Escape From Dementia

Retaining the Mind Series: Book 1 Revision 2

WILLIAM EMMETT WALSH, MD

ISBN-13: 978-1-7346396-1-2 (paperback)

Edited by Peter Bergh
Typeset and Cover Design by www.ebookbook.com

Printed in the United States of America

Other Books by Dr. Walsh

Home Allergies: Don't Let Your Home Make You Sick

Food Allergies: The Complete Guide to Understanding and Relieving Your Food Allergies

The Food Allergy Book: The Foods That Cause You Pain and Discomfort and How to Take Them out of Your Diet

Treating Food Allergy, My Way: Exploring the Most Important Food Allergies, Second Edition

Treating Sinus, Migraine, and Cluster Headaches, My Way: An Allergist's Approach to Headache Treatment

Treating Food Allergy, My Way: Exploring the Most Important Food Allergies

Retaining the Mind: How the Foods We Eat Affect Our Brain

How I Recovered From Dementia

Contents

Chapter 7
Refined Sugar   59

Chapter 8
Citrus Acids   72

Acknowledgments

Many people helped me as I prepared this book, and I am deeply grateful. I thank my family, especially Mary Cecilia, Meredithe, and Bill Jr., who helped me through the many months of preparation. I thank my staff who helped me care for my patients. Thanks to Dr. Bill Hicks for his support, for his care for my patients when I retired, and for the wonderful foreword he has provided. His words once again remind me of how much I miss my patients who also became my friends.

Of supreme importance, thanks to my patients who guided me on my path to understanding the dangers in our modern diet.

Foreword

I first met Dr. Bill Walsh and his wife, Cec, in 2010. I had just completed my Allergy and Immunology fellowship and was ready to start a new career. Dr. Walsh was ready to retire after forty years in private allergy practice in Saint Paul, Minnesota, and I was hoping to step in as the new allergist. The first thing that was evident to me upon walking through the doors of Dr. Walsh's practice was that his patients adored him. They felt listened to, cared for, and validated. His would not be an easy act to follow.

I had the honor of working beside Dr. Walsh in the six months before his retirement. Now, I happily call him a friend. Knowing what I do now, I understand why his patients love him so much. Dr. Walsh's motivation in practicing medicine was never prestige, or money, or notoriety. It was—and remains—the desire to help people. I do my best to bring to my practice the sincere goodwill that his patients have come to expect, though I am no Dr. Walsh. It's been years since he retired, and his patients still ask about him on a regular basis. So often I hear: "What's Dr. Walsh up to?" or "I was miserable until I met Dr. Walsh"—and even "Dr. Walsh was lifesaving."

In short, he is sorely missed by many.

It is not just Dr. Walsh's sincerity that makes him special; it is also his unique medical perspective. He happens to be an allergist whose diet has affected his own health for many years. His personal experience informs the way he thinks about health—his own and others. In this book, he discusses how his views are not always perfectly aligned with what he refers to as "evidence-based medicine," but how they have been profoundly helpful for himself and others, nonetheless.

Perhaps the most special thing that Dr. Walsh does—which is rare not just among doctors but among people everywhere—is truly listen. I don't mean the kind of polite listening with excellent eye contact and nodding at the correct times; I'm talking about listening to hear and listening to learn. His mantra, which I understood within an hour of meeting him, is: Always listen to the patient. It takes a unique and rare blend of humility and self-confidence to sit across from a patient as if you are a pupil. This is something that I've learned from Dr. Walsh that isn't taught well in medical school. Dr. Walsh takes what he learns from his teachers—his patients—and forms patterns and insights.

As you read this book, you will find multiple references to patients whom Dr. Walsh has followed. Many of them may well be those who are in my office today asking about his well-being. Their health improved under his care and, in addition, they felt regarded. It's easy to see from *Retaining the Mind* that Dr. Walsh's interactions have altered his understanding and resulted in rethinking his medical beliefs. So often, as doctors, we try to fit a patient into the confines of what we have been taught. Dr. Walsh is mindful of those confines but continues to be willing to explore outside of them.

Now, after retiring from a successful medical practice, instead of going to the beach, he is driven to share this knowledge in order to help others. He combines his personal experience of food sensitivities with years of listening to thousands of patients to bring you the recommendations in this book.

Much of what is included in this book is not pulled from medical textbooks or journals; rather it is from a doctor who was always been open to learning from his patients. His knowledge and careful attention have afforded him a unique perspective that is new and different. Now he wants to pass this to you.

William Brent Hicks, MD
Board certified in allergy and immunology
Member, American College of Allergy,
Asthma, and Immunology

Introduction

Our Modern Diet Breeds Disease

I have great news. Dementias like Alzheimer's, Parkinson's, and Lewy Body diseases do not have to be lethal. The National Institutes of Health describes dementias as progressive, unstoppable, and deadly: These untreatable diseases continue to destroy the brain until they kill us. This description is no longer accurate for those who understand the dementias and know how to control them. I know this because I have both Alzheimer's and Parkinson's diseases, and I will not let either dementia destroy my mind or kill me.

You may think the dementias are challenging to understand; they are not. They are simple diseases, and my books explain this simplicity. They also examine the Mediterranean Diet that teaches us about the illnesses that arise from our diet and guides us in realizing that our foods make us susceptible to most of our diseases. We will explore the Mediterranean and other diets as we look at diseases and their causes.

You may not believe that our foods and beverages cause deadly diseases, but they can and do cause illnesses. We eat harmful foods and drinks in our daily meals and snacks; no other cause of sickness has the same opportunity to harm us. This frequent exposure to troubling foods makes them destructive and even deadly. However, by carefully choosing our diets, we can control dementia instead of dementia controlling us. By managing dementia, we can recover.

As a medical doctor and board-certified allergist and immunologist, I diagnosed and treated many diseases of our modern diet. I continue to learn about diseases from an excellent teacher, my dementia. In 2015 my dementia controlled me so thoroughly that I lost much of my ability to talk and think. I stopped this disease and reversed it, repairing its damage. By changing my diet, I regained speech and thinking, and I will teach you how to recover your mental alertness.

By following my diet, I feel great! I do not need someone to dress and feed me—I preserved my precious independence. I bring you my *Retaining the Mind* series to give you the same chance to recover. To gain this chance, you only need to try my approach to treatment.

Note: To ensure you are looking at my books from among the William Walsh authors, look for my middle name in my signature, William *Emmett* Walsh, MD.

1

Recovery From Alzheimer's Disease

I Discover That I Have Alzheimer's Disease

As a consultant allergist and immunologist, each year I evaluated and treated hundreds of new patients referred to me by their primary medical caregivers because they suffered illnesses caused by their diet. However, until I retired, I did not realize that the disease I dreaded most was stalking me. Nerve deterioration was destroying my ability to talk and think

My failing mental health forcefully captured my attention when I had the honor to introduce a speaker at a meeting. I had given lectures to referring doctors and the general public for years, and I had enjoyed giving those speeches. I shouldn't have stumbled over a four-minute introduction.

But I did stumble at a meeting where I was scheduled to introduce the speaker. Intact memory is essential for presenting without notes. Speaking before an audience is easy if a speaker is experienced but impossible if the speaker's mind is deteriorating. Unfortunately, my mind was deteriorating. I could not think; I could not speak; I could not give the introduction. I could only sit down! This forced the speaker to stand up and introduce herself. What a disaster! I was humiliated.

That experience made me admit to myself that I was suffering the mental deterioration of Alzheimer's disease. I knew its cause. I knew that I needed to avoid the foods and beverages that cause my nerve deterioration, to follow the same advice that I had given to so many patients. I changed my diet. The results delight me. My mental decline at first slowed and then reversed itself. I am again able to speak to a group. And, in everyday conversation, I can formulate complete sentences.

If I return to eating the offending foods, I again form sentences poorly. If the poor diet choices are limited to a day or two and I hurry back to my diet, eliminating the foods that caused my deterioration, the stumbling sentences disappear after about twenty-four hours.

I hope my story helps you understand the following principle: Avoiding or limiting certain foods can reverse nerve deterioration—including the deterioration of the brain's nerves. These nerves can recover from years of abuse. (Complete recovery may take some years.) The fact that mental deterioration is reversible is the first reason I wrote this book. I will now give a second reason.

A conversation in a restaurant prompted me to return to writing about illnesses caused by our modern diet. I did not need much prompting because it fascinates me to watch the words flow from my mind onto paper, words carrying thoughts that can help people feel well.

One night I was enjoying a pleasant meal in a restaurant

with my friends Mickey and Peter. During our conversation, Mickey asked me what aspect of working with my patients I enjoyed the most. I told her that I enjoyed treating patients who suffered from food sensitivity.

Mickey was surprised at my response and replied, "I thought that food reactions were difficult to diagnose and treat."

"It can be," I replied. "But if you know certain information, diagnosis and treatment is not too difficult."

A Short Introduction to a Confusing Problem

I told Mickey that, during my first years of medical practice, I did not understand why foods make people suffer—or what foods were responsible. I should have known about illness caused by food; after all, I was a fellow of the Mayo Clinic's program in allergy and immunology—an excellent program at an outstanding institution. I had passed the American Board of Allergy and Immunology tests that certified that I was an allergy and immunology specialist. Despite all this preparation, I still did not know why patients suffered symptoms from their diets. I thought these patients must be wrong; food could not be causing their symptoms—wasn't it innocent of the charges? After years of diagnosing and treating food sensitivity in my patients, I discovered they were right: In doubting them, I had been wrong. They had much to teach me.

What My Patients Taught Me

Over the years, my patients told me about foods that caused distressing symptoms like frequent headaches, recurrent diarrhea, persistent constipation, terrible itching, progressive mental deterioration, and many other chronic, miserable symptoms. As I evaluated and treated these patients, I also listened to them as they taught me that they suffered sensitivity to certain foods and beverages.

I was so grateful for this knowledge that I resolved to pass this information on to my patients, their primary doctors, and even those who would never come to me for evaluation. With that as my goal, I eventually published books on people's reactions to their diets.

Unfortunately, most people who suffer from food sensitivity have an incomplete understanding of the diet that causes them so much distress. How can they follow a healthy diet if they do not know which foods to avoid? As I talked to my friends in that restaurant, I realized that better knowledge about our diet's dangers could lead the public to better health. I knew I needed to write again about food sensitivity.

"You Came Back to Life"

My diet slows or defeats many diseases, reducing the alarming cost of medical treatment. We follow this treatment in our own homes, at our dining table. A dear friend best expressed, in a few words, the aim of this book when she reflected on my recovery from Alzheimer's symptoms. She stated: "You came back to life." She was right. Maintaining my ability to think, talk, feed, and clothe myself maintains my independence and re-awakens my life. I want to share that joy with you.

2
The Foods That Cause Dementia

At the most basic level, certain foods cause illnesses because they contain significant amounts of problem chemicals. It is these chemicals in foods that make us sick, not the foods themselves. These chemicals are:

Monosodium glutamate (abbreviated as MSG)
Low-calorie sweeteners
Gluten
Refined sugars
Citrus acids
Lactose

You may already be familiar with the harm attributed to gluten and refined sugar. As you look at the rest of the list, you may ask yourself, "Can these other food chemicals also cause problems?" My answer is: "Yes, in my experience, all of these food chemicals can cause symptoms in people sensitive to them."

If sensitive people could reduce the amount of these

chemicals they consume, these foods would lose their power to cause harm. They would feel well. Even people sensitive to these chemicals react only to consuming excess amounts and tolerate them in lesser amounts. Therefore, sensitive sufferers can avoid harm by avoiding these excesses.

If you share a sensitivity to one or all of these food chemicals, this book will help you identify the foods and beverages that contain excesses of these chemicals. Unfortunately, our modern diet contains high levels of these chemicals, and these levels have entered our diet only recently. They were not part of the diet of our ancestors through countless generations over the many eons that formed our genes. Our ancestors did not eat or drink large amounts of these food chemicals until relatively recent times, a short period in our evolutionary history. In the many millions of years of evolution that programmed our genes to tolerate excesses of some food chemicals and not others, a few thousand years is only a blink of the eye. We are not genetically prepared for our current diet.

Principles Guiding Our Study of Food Sensitivity

Now that you are aware of the suspect food chemicals, let us look at the principles that guide me in my study of food sensitivities:

- The foods themselves do not cause reactions; food chemicals cause the reactions.
- The high levels of chemicals are recent additions to our diets.
- Many people tolerate excessive consumption of these chemicals throughout life.

- Many of us have not developed this tolerance.
- Food-sensitive people tolerate these food chemicals as youths but with age they lose this tolerance.
- These troubling foods cause no symptoms if consumed in reasonable amounts.
- These six diet chemicals are small molecules that cannot cause allergic reactions. (Allergy-causing molecules are larger.)
- Symptoms caused by reactions to these food chemicals usually appear hours to days after eating the foods.
- Reactions to food allergies typically strike as the food is eaten or soon after.
- Minute amounts of food can trigger food allergy symptoms.
- Food sensitivity reactions usually require more significant quantities.
- There are infrequent exceptions to these characteristics.

There is one crucial concept in this list of relationships: We are discussing food sensitivity, not food allergy. The causes of food allergies and food sensitivities differ, and an allergy is far easier to diagnose.

Back to the Restaurant Conversation

Now that you have some idea about what it means to have a sensitivity to food chemicals, let's return to the restaurant and the conversation with Mickey and Peter. I had mentioned that the differences between food allergies and food sensitivities confuse many people, but understanding this distinction helps us understand the distress caused by food.

I told Mickey and Peter that the most common cause of suffering related to food intake is not allergy to foods but food sensitivity—the inability to tolerate large amounts of certain foods common in our diet. I regret that so many people suffer from eating foods that contain these excesses of food chemicals. These foods are good for us and should be included in our diets, just not in such large amounts.

Naming This Food Sensitivity

I find it challenging to think of food sensitivity as a "disease" or an "illness." To me, naming it a disease implies an infection. Calling it an illness or sickness suggests much the same. I believe that the sensitivity to these food chemicals is not an illness, disease, or sickness. Instead, it is a *poisoning* of the body by chemicals in foods. Although calling it an illness, infection, or cancer doesn't sound right, I must use these terms to discuss food sensitivities in this book because they are the terms commonly used. As we examine any one of the six individual food chemicals, I will use the name of that chemical followed by either "sensitivity" or "intolerance" (for example, "citric acid sensitivity" or "citric acid intolerance").

Excesses of these troubling food chemicals occur in both food and beverages. Please be aware that whenever I mention foods, I also mean drinks, although I may not add "and beverages."

To avoid naming all six food chemicals each time I discuss them as a group, I will refer to them as the "aging chemicals" because they age us. They add years to our age.

Sensitivity to this group of food chemicals causes many of the discomforts and disabilities we associate with growing older. These chemicals injure nerves; nerves control our bodies and brains. So, when these chemicals harm and kill our nerves, we experience difficult planning, fading memories, weakening balance, degraded toilet habits, and other difficulties that plague the elderly.

When I consider these diet chemicals' profound effects on our life and behavior as we age, I believe that there is no better name for them than the aging chemicals.

Caution

Although I will be presenting information on dementia in this book, this book will not diagnose your condition—so do not try to make it your doctor. When I was in practice, I could not diagnose my patients' illnesses unless I saw them, questioned them, examined them, and studied the results of any necessary tests. Through this book, I cannot see you, examine you, talk with you, or arrange for tests. Instead, my purpose is to acquaint you with common and harmful conditions that arise from the modern diet through my own experience with dementia. It would be best if you discussed with your caregiver the possibility that you are similarly affected by sensitivity to certain foods.

If you suffer from any diagnosed food allergies, you must continue limiting or avoiding the foods that cause your allergic symptoms while also handling the aging chemicals cautiously. If you suffer from combined food allergy and food sensitivity, your diet choices will be more complicated, and the help of a dietician may be essential to make sure you are eating a healthy diet.

3
Identifying the Aging Chemicals

They Hide From the Sufferer

Food sensitivity hides from the affected person. Affected people typically believe that in the past, the foods that they have tolerated without symptoms cannot cause symptoms today—symptoms like headaches or abdominal distress or dementia. However, this idea is wrong. My patients' stories showed me that foods they tolerated well earlier in life could cause miserable symptoms with age. This increased sensitivity with age happens frequently. Later-in-life sensitivity becomes easier to believe when sufferers realize that, as aging brings many changes such as hair loss and decreased muscle tone, it also brings a lower tolerance to many food chemicals.

Not everybody loses hair or muscle tone with age, and not everybody loses their tolerance to these aging chemicals as they age. But if they lose this tolerance, they must avoid eating excessive amounts of the offending foods, or they suffer.

Another Reason They Hide From the Sufferer

The second reason people fail to realize that their diet makes them ill is that they can eat limited amounts of these chemicals without experiencing symptoms. Often my patients asked me: "But I just ate (or drank) some of it yesterday and had no trouble. Why should it trouble me today?" My answer is, "Yesterday, you did not eat (or drink) enough to trigger your stomach pain and diarrhea (or headaches or forgetfulness), but today you exceeded the amount that you tolerate, and now you suffer. If you abuse your diet for some time, it takes about three days to eliminate from your body the gluten (or other offending chemicals) that you ate. If you stray from your diet for a shorter time, maybe only one meal or one day, the recovery may take only one day. Overindulgence over several days or weeks, even if it is only mild overindulgence, can accumulate sufficient food chemicals in your body to trigger symptoms. Once you suffer symptoms, one to three days on a cautious diet must pass before you can safely return to eating limited amounts of that food."

People suffering from the aging chemicals need to realize that, although as youngsters, they could eat large quantities of foods with these aging chemicals without suffering symptoms, now they are older and can no longer tolerate the same amounts of these foods. Further, they must realize that eating small amounts of these foods without symptoms does not mean that they can eat more significant amounts without suffering. Once they comprehend these factors, this sensitivity has more difficulty hiding from them.

These Chemicals Hide From Doctors

Not only does the impact of these sensitivities hide from affected people, but it also hides from doctors, again for two reasons.

The First Reason They Hide

First, although blood, x-ray, or other tests can diagnose many illnesses, no test can diagnose food sensitivity. An example of a disease that a test can diagnose is celiac disease. I am not discussing celiac disease in this book, even though I will be discussing gluten sensitivity. If you have celiac disease, this is not the book for you—you must follow the treatment for celiac disease, not the treatment I advocate here.

In my years as an allergist/immunologist with a great interest in the immune diseases arising from the diet, I diagnosed and treated hundreds of gluten-sensitive patients. I tested many for celiac disease; only three of my patients had positive tests that diagnose celiac disease. All the rest had sensitivity to the aging chemicals that we discuss here. Although I found celiac disease rarely, I found much food sensitivity. Although I treated impressive numbers of these patients, they are only a tiny fraction of the millions of people suffering from food sensitivities.

The Second Reason They Hide

The second reason the symptoms caused by these food chemicals hide from doctors can be summarized in two terms: "evidence-based medicine" and "medical peer review." "Evidence-based medicine" means that doctors should provide evidence—by using appropriate tests—that the studied patients suffer an identified disease or sickness and are treated with the treatment that clinical trials show to be most effective. "Medical peer review" means that the clinical trials on which doctors base their treatment must be judged valid and reliable by experts in the studied condition. Doctors treating patients affected by the aging chemicals have almost no peer-reviewed clinical trials on which to depend.

These treatment trials are not available because there is no group of patients proven—through recognized laboratory or x-ray tests—to suffer food sensitivity. Unfortunately, developing these tests will be challenging as food sensitivity is food poisoning and challenging to measure. The harmful chemicals are standard parts of the body, not foreign like cyanide or other poisons, and dangerous only when consumed in excess of tolerance. Therefore, doctors have little or no "peer-reviewed," "evidence-based" treatment to follow.

An example of the same frustrating lack of evidence-based treatment exists for the millions of people who suffer the ill-defined pain called *headaches*. The pain itself is difficult to define; there are many causes of headaches, and many of these causes are unidentified. As in food sensitivity, because doctors cannot diagnose the cause of many headaches, peer-reviewed, evidence-based approaches are not available to treat many types of headaches.

This lack of confirmatory testing does not mean that these chemicals cause no pain or suffering or that they plague only a few. Millions suffer pain and distress from these chemicals.

Medical Tests Cannot Diagnose Food Sensitivity

What should the doctor do when a patient is suffering, the cause cannot be diagnosed by tests, and the symptoms are non-specific? If the reason is food sensitivity, the doctor must suspect this problem and advise patients to try a healthy diet. As you pity the patient, also pity doctors who do not understand the problem; they do not know what to do for patients who suffer from these sensitivities.

There is one more consequence to the aging chemicals' ability to hide from doctors: It seriously hampers me in telling you about the specific causes and outcomes of food sensitivities since medical tests cannot diagnose this condition.

It would be different if I were teaching you about an illness that can be tested, like a food allergy identified by skin tests or asthma that pulmonary function tests identify. In these cases, I could tell you the results of clinical trials studying patients with food allergies or asthma. Because tests cannot confirm food sensitivity, I had to use treatment trials by diet change to identify food sensitivity.

Even with this lack of evidence-based diagnosis and treatment, you need to know about food chemical sensitivity to determine whether you suffer from it and how to avoid it. I will use the results of food studies, the clinical experience I gained during my forty years of treating my food-sensitive patients, and the years of treating my own food sensitivity to give you this information.

4

Monosodium Glutamate

The name "monosodium glutamate" signifies an amino acid—glutamic acid (also called glutamate)—where a sodium ion replaces a hydrogen. Glutamic acid is one of the amino acids that form our body's proteins when tightly bonded to other amino acids (for example, our red and white blood cells, muscles). It is one of the amino acids that form organs like the liver, spleen, and brain. These proteins need glutamic acid. It is essential for life and harmless when tightly bound to, or imprisoned within, protein.

In this chapter, we will discuss how breaking apart proteins releases amino acids, including glutamic acid. Once free of its protein prison and combined with sodium, glutamic acid floats freely in water, including the water in our bloodstream, and reaches all parts of our bodies. In this state, this amino acid is "free" glutamic acid, monosodium glutamate, or, simply, MSG.

You need to understand MSG to discover why it is both essential for life and dangerous. Because there is so much information you need to know, I have divided this information into numbered parts.

Part 1: Free Glutamic Acid—A Potent and Worrisome Amino Acid

There is nothing unusual about amino acids floating freely in the bloodstream. Once released from their protein prisons, they travel through the body, doing their work of building and repairing the body's proteins—all innocent, all natural, and all helpful. Except, in certain circumstances, when one of these amino acids—glutamic acid—becomes dangerous.

Its power makes glutamic acid dangerous. When free from its protein prison, glutamic acid serves as a potent neurotransmitter: The nerves use glutamic acid to carry a nerve impulse from one neuron to another, a transmission essential in everyday activity. By using glutamic acid as a nerve stimulator, the brain controls the rest of the body. The stimulations start in our brains and range throughout our bodies traveling from one nerve to another until they activate the nerves that control our arms, legs, tongues, and our sense of taste. Commercially, we add it to our foods and beverages to stimulate the nerves of taste to bring a robust flavor to our diet.

To better understand this process, let's really simplify certain situations where your brain stimulates your nerves to trigger actions. These actions can vary from adding up a grocery bill to covering your nose when you sneeze to running as fast as you can when you see a hungry tiger charging at you. In all these situations, your brain needs to activate specific nerve cells to add up the bill, cover the sneeze, or run like mad.

Your brain must be very selective in which nerves it stimulates. If every time you add up a grocery bill, your nerves prompt you to run full speed through the grocery store, bowling over carts and customers, you will be thrown out of the store by enraged customers or store personnel. Or if you start covering your sneeze instead of running when charged by a tiger, only the tiger will be happy.

If the nerves that start in your brain and end in your leg muscles delivered only powerful stimulation to your running muscles, never relaxing after this stimulation, your leg muscles would go into spasm (similar to having an epileptic seizure). It would prevent you from running, drop you to the ground, and, again, make the tiger happy. To prevent this, your brain's command to run away travels through a network of nerves extending from the brain to the nerves that control the leg muscles. The impulse from the nerve network is alternately commanding specific leg muscles to stretch your legs and then retract them while you run.

Electric Cords and Nerves

The network of nerves is like a network of electrical extension cords. This network has the weakness of extension cords—short-circuiting if the wires, hot with electricity, touch each other. To prevent electric cords from touching each other, plastic insulates extension cords so the hot wires do not touch the surrounding hot wires and cause uncontrolled, dangerous sparking. Like the insulated extension cords, a coating called a myelin sheath insulates nerves from each other, preventing them from sending bursts of wild nerve impulses careening through your convulsing body.

Since nerves can't touch each other, how does a stimulus pass from one nerve to another? A chemical leaps across the spaces between neurons (synapses), from the stimulated nerves to the nerves needing stimulation. The stimulation travels from nerve to nerve until reaching the nerves that extend or retract the leg muscles. By alternatively extending and then retracting your leg muscle, your body moves, allowing you to flee from the tiger.

This chemical has to be a potent nerve stimulator (neuro stimulant) telling the nerves of the legs to run, strong enough to force the nerves of the leg to obey. Unfortunately, a chemical so overpowering—so commanding—carries the danger, in certain situations, of overstimulating and damaging nerves, thereby becoming a neurotoxin.

The most common chemical used by the body to stimulate nerves is the neuro-stimulating amino acid glutamic acid—MSG. Its decisive action can be hazardous to nerves if not rapidly cleared away from the space between the nerves before it harms the nerve.

Once the glutamic acid clears from the space between two nerves, this nerve stimulation ends very quickly. If this nerve is stimulating a muscle that makes the leg extend, ending the stimulus allows the extending muscle to relax while another nerve activates the muscle that contracts the leg. This quick extension/contraction powers the running that helps evade the tiger.

When Glutamic Acid Harms

Unfortunately, the "washing out" of the MSG from the synapse may—and in many people does—weaken as they age. The weakness turns excess MSG intake from only mildly annoying nerves to injuring them, from neurostimulator to neurotoxin. I am using *toxic* and *toxins* to indicate poisons produced naturally by living things. A poisonous substance can stimulate mildly or severely. Once the body loses its ability to swiftly remove MSG from the synapse, the punishing symptoms suffered by people sensitive to the excess MSG arise.

Unfortunately, in MSG-sensitive people, the mechanism that removes the glutamic acid from the nerve synapse weakens and can fail. Many doctors and scientists believe that this is one of the processes that damage the brain in stroke and Alzheimer's disease. It may also be a cause of epileptic seizures. This failure to clear out the synapses allows excess glutamic acid to accumulate, and large numbers of calcium ions enter the nerve cell, bulging out the cell and harming it.

In short, glutamic acid, MSG, can be dangerous.

A Note of Explanation

Before continuing our discussion about MSG, I want to acknowledge that the companies that produce the food flavoring, MSG, probably believe it causes no harm. I also recognize that it is a natural and effective flavor enhancer. The FDA considers the addition of MSG to foods to be "generally recognized as safe," but I cannot agree. In excess, it is not safe for those sensitive to the nerve damage inflicted by MSG.

Why This Discussion About Glutamic Acid?

MSG plays an essential role in keeping us alive—without it, our nerves would communicate poorly, and our ancestors would have been fine feasts for lions, tigers, bears, and other predators. However, in many people, the good that MSG does is overshadowed by its harm. MSG sensitivity explains why so many people suffer a multitude of painful and disabling illnesses.

I am a specialist in food allergy, sensitivity, and the immunology of disease. If you understand the information about MSG that I am presenting, it also will help you know the other aging chemicals.

Now let's look at the symptoms that can affect MSG-sensitive people.

Part 2: Symptoms Caused by MSG

In this section, I will use three sources of information to tell you about the symptoms caused by MSG. First, I will tell you about the symptoms I, as an Alzheimer sufferer, experience when I overindulge in food or drink flavored with MSG. Second, I will tell you about the symptoms suffered by a dear friend who first alerted me to the potential harm caused by MSG. Third, I will discuss how MSG troubled many of the patients who came to me for evaluation and treatment.

I have already told you that the aging chemicals affect me; I have reacted to them for many years. I know my symptoms well; they helped me understand the thousands of food-sensitive patients who came to me for diagnosis and treatment. Because I shared their symptoms, within a few minutes of visiting with my food-sensitive patients, I knew why they suffered—and I could fully sympathize with them.

By the way, even though my patients benefited from my experiences with the aging chemicals—and I was pleased that they did benefit—I would rather be resistant to the neurotoxin symptoms of MSG. If I knew how to cure it, I would heal myself today and go back to eating a "normal" diet that includes all the fine-tasting foods I must avoid.

My Symptoms

Sleep Disturbance

My most irritating and persistent symptom is sleep disturbance. It comes in two varieties. If I eat a meal with a gross excess of MSG, I cannot sleep for forty-eight hours. Typically, after two sleepless nights spent looking at my bedroom ceiling, I renew my determination to follow my diet strictly. That resolution lasts for weeks until another delicious meal full of MSG stares up at me from my plate, and my weak willpower tempts me into eating it. This cheating, of course, is followed by another two nights without sleep—and another resolution to avoid this flavoring chemical.

The next variety of sleep disturbance arises when I eat or drink a slight excess of MSG, much less than the gross excess of the meal that brings the forty-eight-hour sleeplessness. All of the aging chemicals can be eaten in small amounts by sensitive people. After all, many of these chemicals reside in acceptable foods, are part of our bodies, are necessary for us to continue living, and small amounts typically do not cause adverse symptoms. Eating or drinking more than these well-tolerated amounts can bring uncomfortable symptoms.

A slight excess of MSG affects my sleep, waking me after four hours of light sleep feeling tired because my sleep was not refreshing, making me wish I could sleep longer. If I avoid this slight excess of MSG for a few days, I return to enjoying a longer and more refreshing sleep. I have found that many of my patients share this four-hour sleep pattern, and I feel confident that this pattern is a sign of MSG sensitivity.

More recent—but far more problematic—symptoms are the memory loss and difficulty speaking I have described in Chapter 1. As MSG interferes with sleep and degrades speech, it also damages memory, making anyone afflicted by this mental deterioration horribly worried.

Diarrhea Followed by Constipation

Of lesser distress to me, although not without annoyance, are bouts of diarrhea and constipation that follow eating or drinking excess MSG. Typically, diarrhea appears hours after MSG excess—up to twenty-four hours later. The cramping of diarrhea subsides after several hours, followed by multiple days of constipation that, at times, can be uncomfortable. The whole process lasts for about three days, after which, if I watch my diet, my bowel movements return to their usual pattern.

I believe that MSG is a significant cause of this alternating constipation and diarrhea. In other sensitive people, reducing the amount of MSG in the diet returns the stool pattern to normal. However, if susceptible people are unaware that they are sensitive to MSG and continue to consume MSG, they will continue to suffer an uncomfortable stool pattern. That is what I experienced before I realized that the source of my chronic constipation arose from my diet and that it returns when I stray too far from my diet.

Many of my patients sensitive to the aging food chemicals suffer similar bouts of constipation and diarrhea, suggesting that food sensitivity is a common cause of these symptoms.

Bloating and Weight Gain

I can also tell when my diet makes me bloat. My belt feels tight and forms an uncomfortable band across my waist; I do not feel this uncomfortable tightness if I avoid the aging chemicals. Further, my bathroom scale shows a two-to-five-pound gain when I consume an excess of these chemicals and weight loss if I avoid them. The weight gain ends with increased urination when I avoid MSG for a few days, pointing to fluid accumulation or edema as the cause of the bloating. Similar bloating afflicts many food-sensitive patients. We discussed the sleeplessness, memory loss, difficulty speaking, bloating, and constipation/diarrhea caused by the aging chemicals, including MSG. Now let's discuss another common symptom, a friend's very painful symptom.

My Friend John's Symptoms

John was an artist, a man whose friendship my wife and I treasured for years. We often vacationed together with John and his wife, and he gave his time as an art mentor for our young son. Thus, it deeply troubled me when my good friend told me about his severe pain. I still remember his description of the pain.

John said, "Bill, this past week, my cluster headaches returned. They return several times a year, and when they return, they often stay for several weeks. Pain waves make me bang my head against a wall to try to take my mind away from the pain."

"John, your headaches are that severe?"

"Yes, my recent attack struck about two hours after a meal, and I believe that the pain came from a sausage I ate before the pain started."

"Did you find out the ingredients of the sausage?"

"No, but will you call the restaurant and find out the ingredients?" I agreed to call for a good reason: If I could identify the cause of John's headaches—and if a food caused them—it might give me a clue into how foods cause headaches. I called the restaurant and found that the only suspicious ingredient in the sausage was MSG.

This conversation started my interest in MSG and its relationship to headaches. As long as John avoided MSG, his headaches became fewer and less painful—but they returned when he again allowed MSG into his diet.

Cluster Headaches

To give you an idea of the power of MSG in causing severely painful headaches, let's examine John's headaches. John suffered cluster headaches, headaches that strike in a "cluster" of episodes, usually without warning, and usually after weeks or months of being free from headaches. They return daily—sometimes several times in a day—and last anywhere from minutes to hours. They usually bring excruciating pain in or around one eye but can strike anywhere about the face, neck, and shoulders.

Typically, during a cluster headache, one eye reddens and tears run from the eye, the skin surrounding the eye swells and reddens, the eyelid droops, and the eye feels like something pushed it out of its socket. At the same time, the nose stuffs up, the face reddens, and sweat blankets the face, and the sufferer moves restlessly. The pain hurts so much that it feels like a hot poker stuck in the eye. (No wonder John bangs his head against a wall to distract him from the pain.)

My Patients' Symptoms

John's experience prompted me to ask my patients if they suffer headaches and, if they said they did, I asked them to watch their diet to see if MSG causes their headaches.

In my practice, each year, for many years, hundreds of new patients consulted me for evaluation and treatment. Many of these patients suffered headaches. The headaches were mainly migraine headaches, with smaller numbers suffering cluster headaches. Through following my advice, many of my patients discovered that eating MSG-flavored foods caused their pain. This response by my patients suggests that in the population at large (not just among my patients), MSG could be bringing tormenting headaches to millions of people.

Part 3: What Our Symptoms Tell Us About MSG

Example: Cluster Headaches

The stories I related above teach us much about the aging chemicals. John's headaches are typical of cluster headaches: His symptoms strongly indicate that stimulation of the trigeminal nerve, the chief sensory nerve of the face, causes the headache pain. This nerve pain refocuses our attention on free glutamic acid (MSG), a potent nerve stimulator (neuro-stimulator) which, when not properly cleared away from the nerve, becomes a nerve toxin (neurotoxin).

Example: Common Migraine Headaches

My experience with migraine sufferers also tells me (and many other doctors agree) that arteries beneath the scalp cause migraine pain. In the form of "common migraine head-aches," these headaches bring intense, throbbing pain to the head, often accompanied by nausea, vomiting, and extreme sensitivity to light and sound.

Scientists are unsure of the causes of common migraine headaches, but the throbbing pain suggests that the pulsating or throbbing of the arteries in the head must be involved. The head has a rich supply of arteries that travel around the head, intimately accompanied by nerves. A coating called the *neurovascular bundles* (neuro refers to nerves, while vascular indicates blood vessels) encases the nerves and blood vessels.

Nerves control the expansion and constriction of blood vessels; damage to the nerves by MSG may exaggerate this expansion of the arteries of the head, causing swollen blood vessels.

Now imagine arteries carrying blood from the heart banging against the nerves they travel with—and these nerves are damaged by overstimulation by the excess MSG in our diet. Throbbing of these nerves by the artery causes a banging, pulsating pain like a swinging door repeatedly closing on a trapped finger. The afflicted suffer a throbbing migraine headache. Ouch!

Damaged nerves cry for relief; pain is the only cry they can make. The pain of migraine headaches may be our bodies begging us to stop all this MSG.

Examples: Basilar and Familial Hemiplegic Migraines

These two forms of migraine headaches point to the interaction of nerves and arteries in the neurovascular bundles and how this interaction causes head pain. Pain from *a basilar migraine* arises from an artery in the base of the brain, in the brainstem, caused by a constriction of blood vessels that limit blood flow to the brain.

An "aura"—a group of sensations such as dizziness, double vision, peculiar odors, and lack of coordination—often alerts the sufferer ten- to forty-five minutes before the headache starts. Inappropriate stimulation of the nerves that control sight, smell, and body coordination causes the aura. Combined with the headache's pulsating pain, the aura demonstrates how the arteries and nerves can team up to cause throbbing headaches.

At least in certain conditions, gene mutation can also cause symptoms involving neurostimulators like MSG. *Hemiplegic migraines* (hemiplegia means paralysis of one side of the body) are similar to basilar migraines because the symptoms of the two are similar except that muscle weakness accompanies the attacks of hemiplegic migraines.

The value of putting hemiplegic migraines under our magnifying glass is that the cause of this type of migraine headache is known—and it is genetic: Mutations in specific genes (CACNA1A, ATP1A2, SCN1A, and PRRT2) cause it. Therefore, in addition to aging, gene mutation influences migraine headaches.

Scientists have discovered the function of these mutant genes, and it shifts our attention back to glutamic acid. These mutated genes provide instructions for making proteins that help neurostimulators like MSG pass their stimulation to the next nerve. (Remember that the leading neurotransmitter in the brain is glutamic acid/MSG.) Because of the inadequate work of these mutated genes, the body only poorly flushes MSG from around nerves, making the possessors of these genes susceptible to the harmful effects of MSG and especially susceptible to migraine headaches.

Headaches and Dementia

Perhaps, in aging people, similar gene mutations or constricted basilar arteries—present since birth and waiting to be triggered—predispose to dementia. If so, these mutations and constrictions hide well because researchers studying aging people still seek them. If they are present, and researchers could find them, these researchers would finally possess the diagnostic tests they desire to perform the peer-reviewed clinical trials that would better identify the cause of headaches and dementia. That would be wonderful.

In the meantime, we can apply what we have learned from basilar and hemiplegic migraines about MSG-damaged nerves causing headaches to understand their participation in causing symptoms other than headaches. The chronic symptoms of diarrhea and constipation that trouble so many people, including me, can be caused by MSG irritation of the nerves in the intestine.

Poor sleep is another condition explained by MSG-irritated nerves. Areas that control sleep/wakefulness run through the brain, from the spinal cord to the cerebral cortex (in other words, from the bottom to the top of the brain). The sleeplessness that occurs after excess MSG eating—and the four-hour broken sleep pattern resulting from continuous MSG eating—must be caused by this irritation of brain nerve cells in these wake/sleep areas of the brain.

There may be those who object to these conclusions, who claim that MSG cannot affect the brain. Let them call me at two o'clock in the morning after I eat an MSG meal while I lie awake looking at the ceiling, and I will tell them what I think of their objections.

Part 4: Why Avoiding MSG Inhibits Symptoms of Aging

So far, in our discussion of MSG, I have been giving you enough information to realize that you should consume less MSG if you are sensitive to it. To consume less, you must avoid many foods and beverages you enjoy. Your reward for this avoidance is a resurrection of damaged nerves.

You might enjoy a return to restful sleep. Many scientific studies show that a lack of restful sleep damages the health of the body and hastens mental decline. In other words: Poor sleep ages your brain—and your body.

I dread aging; I hate losing my freedom and do not want to start depending on the care of others or to need help, even in my toilet care. I want to continue to enjoy the white of the winter snow, the planting and growing of flowers, and the writing of books. The fear of accelerated aging scared me so much that I resolved to change my diet when I found myself sinking into mental deterioration. I knew that only in this way could I avoid these humiliating experiences.

If you also want to live independently, enjoy nature's beauty, and not live in a memory unit, you must be careful of your diet. With a careful diet, we all have a great chance to maintain the independence and self-respect you and I desperately desire.

If MSG Is so Dangerous, Why Is It Widely Used in Our Diet?

MSG stimulates nerves, including the nerves in the taste buds on the surface of the mouth, tongue, and throat. This stimulation does not confer a particular flavor on foods but accentuates the delicious taste of any food. This pleasing sensation makes almost any food taste great. I can usually tell when a food or drink contains high levels of MSG because it is exquisite: This warns me that imminent poor sleep, uncomfortable abdominal distress, and slowing of the brain will make me regret eating it. Most of the time, I do not eat beyond the first bite because my willpower wins. Unfortunately, as I mentioned, sometimes my resolve sleeps (and I don't).

Part 5: Identifying the Sources of MSG

Plants Altered by Farmers to Have High Levels of Free Glutamic Acid

Foods altered by farmers to contain higher levels of free glutamic acid taste much better than foods from original, unaltered plants, which have lower levels of this amino acid. Over many centuries, farmers picked out the better-tasting foods to replant, steadily improving the food's taste while also increasing its content of the free MSG that confers the improved taste. Today, many of our "natural" foods are highly modified from the way they originally appeared, are no longer in their genuinely natural forms, and contain increased levels of MSG.

MSG-sensitive people can eat these "natural" foods but must do so with some caution, eating and drinking only as much of these MSG-containing foods and beverages as they can tolerate. A list of these foods is given below.

Corn

Known in much of the world as "maize," its original form seems to have been a grass-like plant domesticated (meaning that it was used in farming and changed at the genetic level through generations of selective planting) by native farmers in prehistoric times, between 7,000 and 12,000 years ago. More recently, extensive genetic modification resulted in many varieties of today's good-tasting, high-MSG corn.

Twenty percent of the protein content of corn is glutamic acid—much of it imprisoned in protein and harmless, but some not imprisoned and free to be absorbed quickly into the body. This high glutamic acid content suggests that much of corn's glutamic acid is in the form of MSG, part of the reason people react to corn. I react, and many of my patients share my sensitivity to corn. As with all increased-MSG foods, a limited amount of corn should not cause distress in people sensitive to glutamic acid. The amount of corn tolerated differs from individual to individual. Watching for symptoms when consuming it can suggest the tolerance level. Of course, people *allergic* to corn should altogether avoid it. (Corn, including corn on the cob, seems to be better tolerated by boiling the kernels until soft and the boiling water then discarded.)

Quinoa

Quinoa belongs to the goosefoot family of plants, and although it contains gluten, it is not the type of gluten found in wheat, rye, barley, and oats. Thus, in theory, quinoa should be a good substitute for these grains for gluten-sensitive people.

However, I believe that similar to corn, it can cause symptoms in MSG-sensitive people. I have prepared quinoa for myself numerous times, varying every preparation step I could think of, including boiling time. Following every meal, I suffered a sleepless night—a symptom of a food that will bother food-sensitive people. Because of my experience, I cannot advise quinoa for people sensitive to MSG.

Tomatoes and Potatoes

When tomatoes and potatoes were domesticated is unknown, but they were already being cultivated in Mexico over 2,000 years ago. Tomatoes and potatoes were initially derived from the same plant, of the solanum family, with tomatoes growing among the leaves of the plant and potatoes growing underground in the roots.

Tomatoes and potatoes contain a high level of the flavor enhancer, free glutamic acid, its sister amino acid aspartic acid, and citric acid. The act of processing tomato products concentrates both the MSG and citrus content of tomatoes.

It is best not to indulge too heavily in tomatoes, especially processed tomatoes, and to use limited amounts of sliced tomato instead of processed tomato if you suffer from the aging chemicals. Eating potatoes at frequent meals also allows the accumulation in your body of excess MSG, aspartic acid, and citrus acids.

Peanut
Archeologists have dated the oldest specimens of peanuts, found in Peru to about 7,600 years ago. Since that time, the extended period of cultivation allowed farmers to plant the peanuts that tasted best continually. The peanuts that tasted best were those with high levels of free glutamic acid. Avoid or limit your intake of peanuts and peanut-containing products.

Foods That Naturally Contain High Levels of Free Glutamic Acid

Fungus and Yeast Foods
Fungi, also referred to as yeasts and mold, are single-celled or many-celled organisms extensively used in food and drink preparations. Baker's yeast causes bread to rise; other yeasts ferment alcoholic beverages, and others assist in making products such as soy sauce, sake, miso, and tempeh. Fungus and yeast have naturally high levels of free glutamic acid in their bodies and are often added to foods to improve the flavor of the foods.

Mushrooms
Some strains of fungus living in the ground extend these fleshy, spore-bearing fruiting bodies above ground to release into the air the spores that develop into new fungus. As they have a high content of free glutamic acid, avoid them and the foods they season.

Algae
Seaweed is the common name for a grass-like sea plant made up of multicellular marine algae. Seaweed has been used for

years to flavor foods. The reason for this improved taste was unknown until scientists extracted MSG from the seaweed and identified it as the flavor enhancer that causes such a remarkably improved taste in foods.

Extracts from seaweed, named "agar" and "carrageenan," are used in food manufacturing to keep mixed ingredients from separating and give foods a smooth texture. Commercial preparations of agar and carrageenan may contain free amino acids, including both aspartic and glutamic acid. Even though experts regard both amino acids as harmless, you should avoid or limit foods containing agar and carrageenan if you have issues with MSG sensitivity.

Joanne K. Tobacman, associate professor of clinical medicine at the University of Chicago, has studied carrageenan and is concerned. She notes that carrageenan has been used in laboratory animals to induce inflammation, the same chronic inflammation active in heart disease, Alzheimer's, Parkinson's, and cancer. Many food products contain carrageenan and, depending on the foods you include in your diet, your exposure may be higher than you think.

You will find seaweed or its derivatives, carrageenan and agar, on the list of ingredients of many foods made from milk, like yogurt, ice cream, and cottage cheese. They are found in jelly, chocolate, and salad dressing and in pie filling and processed meats, where food manufacturers use them as a fat substitute. Please read the label of any of these foods carefully and decide whether you want to consume them.

How Fermentation, Autolysis, and Proteolysis Provide MSG

I have pointed out that mold and yeast ferment alcoholic beverages, such as beer, wine, whiskey, and soy products, such as tofu and soy sauce, and how this fermentation increases free glutamic acid content (MSG). We can add bacteria to the list of organisms used in fermentation, especially in cheese creation. These foods contain protein, and the fermentation process splits apart the protein, freeing the bound amino acids, including glutamic acid.

The microorganisms doing the fermenting also contain significant levels of free glutamic acid inside their cells. When these microorganisms die and disintegrate, they release their content of potent digestive enzymes, and these enzymes further degrade proteins to amino acids—a process called self-digestion or *autolysis*. In this way, autolysis increases the content of free amino acids, including free glutamic acid in the form of MSG, in the food. Food labels note this increased content as "autolyzed yeast extract."

The breaking down of protein into amino acids by an outside source is called *proteolysis*. The chemicals that promote proteolysis are present in many organisms, including yeast, bacteria, plants, and animals. Several commercial products use proteolysis to tenderize tough meat fibers using papain from the papaya, bromelain from pineapple, and actinidin from the kiwi fruit. If you suffer from MSG sensitivity, it is best to avoid meat tenderized with these proteolytic chemicals, as the levels of MSG may be more than you can tolerate.

Every fermented product contains MSG. The higher the original protein content in the food being fermented, the higher the MSG content in the fermented food or beverage. Because cereal grains such as wheat and barley are mainly carbohydrates and contain lesser amounts of protein, they release less MSG than protein-heavy milk or soybeans. High-protein content is why food manufacturers use soy and milk proteins in the industrial production of MSG. Fermentation and autolysis also explain why cheese, especially well-aged cheeses, contains so much MSG. When you think of cheese, think of MSG.

Products With High Levels of Free Glutamic Acid Because of Hydrolysis

Hydrolysis is the breaking apart of protein by boiling it in special solutions, thus freeing glutamic acid from the protein and turning it into free MSG. The freed MSG is then collected and added to foods that do not contain large quantities of MSG. (A note: Hydrolysis is often confused with "hydrogenation." Hydrogenation, however, happens to fats and oils, not proteins, and is not examined in this book.)

Check the list of ingredients on any food to see if a "hydrolyzed protein" (such as hydrolyzed soy or milk protein) is added to the food product you are considering buying. If so, don't buy it.

Hydrolysis also breaks down the protein in meat into amino acids, resulting in gelatin rich in the glutamic acid in the animal protein. So you should probably also avoid products containing gelatin.

Food processors put MSG on the list of ingredients on the label if they use it in its pure form. However, they do not need to note it on the label if they add it in the form of a product that already contains large amounts of MSG such as hydrolyzed protein, autolyzed yeast, Parmesan cheese, or "natural flavoring." This kind of labeling is a common practice, which is why you must know these sources of MSG to avoid eating and drinking them.

Products That Are Concentrated MSG

The final source of MSG in the diet is the glutamic acid manufactured by hydrolysis and autolysis, combined with sodium, calcium, or magnesium, and then dried. When you see monosodium glutamate on the label, you know that the food manufacturer is honest about what the food contains. You can applaud them for their honesty, but you still should not buy the product.

Part 6: Listing MSG on Food Labels

Having discussed how MSG enters our diet, let us look at the following lists I developed as I identified the foods that caused my patients' symptoms, which also affect me. I also included information found on many websites.

Avoid foods with the following ingredients. Any one of these ingredients on the label means free glutamic acid:

- monosodium glutamate
- monopotassium glutamate
- calcium glutamate
- monoammonium glutamate
- magnesium or sodium glutamate

The following foods and beverages are likely to include excess free glutamic acid, and it is best to avoid them.

- Any fermented food or beverage, including:
  - bean-based manufactured products (soy sauce, tofu, soy milk, etc.)
  - manufactured dairy products (cheese, yogurt, etc.)
  - processed fruit-based products (wine, brandy, etc.)
  - processed grain-based products (alcoholic beverages such as beer, whiskey, etc.)
- Any food or beverage containing autolyzed ingredients, including:
  - yeast
  - yeast extract
  - yeast food
  - yeast nutrient
  - torula
  - brewer's yeast
- Any food or beverage containing hydrolyzed ingredients, including any kind of plant or vegetable protein
- Any food containing enzymes or proteases
- Any food or beverage containing protein altered in any way, including:
  - protein-fortified
  - calcium caseinate or sodium caseinate
  - gelatin
  - meat tenderized with papain, bromelain, or actinidin
  - soy protein, soy protein concentrate, or soy protein isolate

- o textured protein
- o whey protein, whey protein concentrate, or wheat protein isolate

If a Food Label Contains These Ingredients, Avoid or Limit Them in Your Diet

- Any flavors or "flavoring", including natural flavor that does not identify the source of the flavoring (remember MSG is a natural flavoring)
- Any food or beverage labeled ultra-pasteurized
- Any malted or sprouted seed, including barley malt or almond milk
- Bouillon and broth
- Pectin
- Unidentified seasonings
- Stock

Natural Foods That Should Be Avoided or Limited in Your Diet

The following natural foods are also high in free glutamic acid, so you should minimize their use in your diet:

- Seaweed (known as kelp and other names) and its products carrageenan and agar
- Lightly cooked corn and corn products, including corn syrup
- Peanuts and peanut products
- Quinoa
- Tomatoes especially concentrated tomato products

Part 7: Summary

In my allergy practice, I found that my MSG patients who overindulge in this flavoring chemical suffer distressing body and mind symptoms. Therefore, for them, following a healthy diet is a blessing and not a curse. By reducing the amount of MSG they consume, they relieve chronic symptoms. They enjoy restful sleep and awaken refreshed. I share these experiences.

Of secondary—but still pleasing—importance: After years of hammering taste buds with MSG, avoiding it awakens the taste buds to the tremendous but subtle flavors in natural foods. For example, the crunching sensation of eating celery is pleasant; now, with recovering nerves of taste, we enjoy flavors in celery not experienced when MSG damaged our nerves. Without excess MSG in our diet, the flavors in meat, vegetable, and fruit awaken our sense of taste delightfully.

We do not need to eliminate MSG completely. We need only to reduce our consumption to the amount we tolerate. Unfortunately, how much MSG we can handle cannot be predicted; we must develop a sense of how much MSG-flavored food we can allow in our diet. This amount will most likely be different from the tolerance of our brother, our best friend, and our neighbor across the street.

To understand this, remember that, as we age, many of our genes also age and the switches that control the genes' power progressively weaken these genes. These are the genes and switches that allow us to tolerate MSG. The switches dim the actions of genes like a dimmer switch reduces the light in a dining room. Similarly, our ability to consume MSG depends on the competence of the genes that regulate MSG metabolism.

If you are sensitive to MSG, even though you do not need to eliminate MSG from your diet completely, you still must be careful of how much you consume. Remember that the effects of excess MSG may last for three days—it takes three days to eliminate the excess from your body. If you eat small quantities of MSG-containing foods for two to three consecutive days, the MSG in the meal on the third day may combine with the MSG from previous meals to bring you headaches, diarrhea, flawed thinking, and other symptoms. It is best to prevent these symptoms by following a low-MSG diet.

Food-sensitive people should consume alcohol in moderation and understand that even small amounts of alcohol add to the total consumption of MSG.

As for me, I dread the onset of the mental deterioration that can accompany aging. I know that any foods that contain the aging chemicals injure and destroy nerves and hasten the start of this horrible deterioration. Any day that I consume a diet low in these chemicals is a day when I resist aging my brain and my body.

It is never too late to reduce the amount of MSG in your diet. You can recover much of your youth, the ability to think, and the gift of remembering. You now know my story, a story that shows that recovery is possible and of that, I am an excellent example. Just do not wait too long to start.

5

Low-Calorie Sweeteners

In this discussion of low-calorie sweeteners (LCS), I will use aspartic acid as a representative of the LCS mainly because it is the sweetener that my patients most used and that I know best. Like glutamic acid, aspartic acid is one of the body's amino acids.

Once my diet relieved my patients' headaches, I did not further investigate the effect of each LCS on symptoms. I could not have undertaken these studies if I had wanted to; my patients would not have agreed to trial doses of different types of LCS to see which brought back their headaches—and I would never have asked them to do so.

So, if I am unkind to any LCS suppliers that do not cause symptoms, I sincerely apologize. But, for our discussion, I will use aspartic acid to discuss the reactions to the LCSs in our diet.

Aspartic Acid Is Related to MSG

When we eat foods, our digestive systems break down the food proteins into the amino acids that make up these proteins. Then, we consume these separated amino acids and use them to form the proteins in all our various structures, organs, and bloodstream components. Like glutamic acid, aspartic acid is not only an essential component of our proteins; it also—like MSG—is a neurostimulator and, in excess, a neurotoxin.

Most of what I discuss about free glutamic acid (MSG) also applies to aspartic acid, with specific differences, mainly concerning the ability of these amino acids to harm sensitive sufferers.

If we compared the harm caused by excess MSG with the damage caused by excess aspartic acid, MSG's power for injury is much greater than that of aspartic acid. If aspartic acid shared our drive and ambitions, it would detest comparison to MSG. Aspartic acid may desire a role as necessary as MSG, but it lacks some of MSG's ability to hide from us.

MSG powerfully stimulates and damages nerves. Aspartic acid probably has this same ability, but unlike MSG, it does not hide in the diet under many different names. If food manufacturers add it to a food or drink, they acknowledge its presence on the label; you know when you are consuming it. The name of the food we eat and the beverage we drink typically signifies the presence of an LCS, a name such as "diet soda" or "low-calorie ice cream." While glutamic acid serves as the most common neurotransmitter and neurotoxin, aspartic acid serves a less critical role.

Aspartic Acid in the Diet

To sweeten foods and drinks, food producers use aspartic acid in the form of aspartame, a combination of the amino acids aspartic acid and phenylalanine, with the trade names NutraSweet, Equal, and others. They sweeten many foods and drinks, including chewing gum, dessert mixes, frozen desserts, pudding, soft drinks, and yogurt. They also are available in dry form in tabletop sweeteners. Even some cough drops and vitamins contain aspartame.

Is Aspartame Safe?

Many people who speak for aspartame believe it to be safe and many studies have examined its safety. These studies have concluded that it does not cause headaches, seizures, Alzheimer's disease, Parkinson's disease, lupus, or multiple sclerosis. Further, no research has identified dangerous health consequences of aspartame.

I Disagree

My experience tells me that aspartame is not safe for patients sensitive to the aging chemicals. My patients suffering headaches pointed to aspartame as a cause of their headaches. Many of these patients came to me already knowing that LCSs such as those found in diet drinks set off painful headaches. Others were unaware of this source of pain but learned about it when I asked them to remove these foods from their diets. Removing them gave them great relief. Freeing them from their headache pain served as a sign to me that my patients suffering from LCS also suffered from sensitivity to the aging chemicals and told me that I must ask them to be very careful of all the aging chemicals.

This experience in headache control prompted me to write about the food chemicals in my book *Treating Sinus, Migraine and Cluster Headaches, My Way.* Once they understood the headache causes that lurk in their homes and environmental allergens, once I told them about food sensitivity and counseled them on their diets, I could relieve many of their headaches.

Aspartic Acid in Natural Foods

I become more and more convinced that what we call *natural* foods—foods such as wheat, corn, apples, and citrus fruits—have been extensively modified over thousands of years by their growers' efforts and are, in fact, genetically altered. Though I will continue to use the term *natural* to differentiate unprocessed foods from processed foods, in my mind, the exact meaning of natural is unclear.

Nature uses both aspartic and glutamic acid in the proteins to make our foods. However, the amount of aspartic acid in natural foods is markedly lower than the amount of glutamic acid. Glutamic acid usually makes up about ten percent of the proteins in foods. In corn, milk, and soy, its level reaches about twenty percent; in gluten, it reaches an even higher level suggesting that farmers extensively modified corn, soy, and gluten from this probable ten-percent glutamic acid level of the original ancestral plants.

The story is much different with aspartic acid. It reaches its peak level at a little over ten percent of protein in alfalfa and corn. In wheat, its concentration is low—only about six percent. I wondered why farmers did not modify these foods to increase their aspartic acid content. I found the answer in bodybuilders' comments about using aspartic acid as a supplement to increase the efficiency of exercising. Those who commented on its taste described it as being unpleasant, even "awful." Being practical and intelligent, farmers did not force more aspartic acid into their crops because there was no advantage to having more of this amino acid than the amount initially there.

If aspartic acid wants to be the kingpin neurostimulator and neurotoxin, dethroning glutamic acid, it couldn't. It remains a wannabe.

Where Aspartic Acid May Be Important

In our discussion of glutamic acid, I noted that it is not the bound glutamic acid in protein that causes symptoms but the glutamic acid freed from protein and freely dispersed by the bloodstream. It is the same with glutamic acid's close relative, aspartic acid.

Besides being added to processed foods, where aspartic acid appears on the label, this water-soluble amino acid also has significant levels in sprouting seeds. Unfortunately, these sprouting seeds include such foods as otherwise healthy quinoa, rice, and corn.

In the process of sprouting, the seed releases both glutamic and aspartic acids from their prisons in protein, converting them into free amino acids. These same free amino acids affect people sensitive to the aging food chemicals. I urge you to watch your intake of these seed foods, confining them to the amount you can tolerate without symptoms.

June 17, 1985
Dear Doctor Walsh:

With this [letter] I want to describe the problems I have had when I've had [*a low-calorie dessert flavored with aspartame*]. The first time, I suffered a reaction—when it first came out—which gave me a terrible headache soon after eating it. This headache did not get any better with aspirin or Tylenol.

[In] the second episode, last month, [I] reacted after only five sips of diet soda. I got shortness of breath, cold sweat, fast heart, and very panicky. These effects wore off after about two hours.

Talking with my neighbor, who is now pregnant, I found out that her OB doctor recommended not drinking anything flavored with aspartame.

A Patient's Symptoms

I asked a patient to write this letter (altered to respect her privacy) describing her experiences with LCSs. She later discovered that she also reacted to corn by developing hives of her cheeks and to MSG with diarrhea.

Without a doubt, my patient suffers from a food allergy and a sensitivity to LCSs. Both MSG and aspartame, two of the aging food chemicals, cause her headaches. Her letter describes a symptom afflicting many patients, headaches with LCS, and also indicates that many sensitive people are aware of the cause of their sensitivity to LCS. It was these patients who taught me so much about food sensitivity.

Helping My Patients

In patients who self-diagnosed so accurately, I could not add to their knowledge of the LCSs. I helped them by expanding their understanding of the other aging food chemicals that cause similar symptoms. Further, when talking to patients who suffer these reactions, I made sure that they knew that a food allergy could cause headaches similar to those caused by the aging food chemicals.

The author of this letter has since tested positive for a corn allergy, so she watches to see if corn causes her any additional distress. Using the above clues in planning her diet helped prevent her headaches.

The Flight or Fight Reaction

Although her letter is short, it contains other excellent information. Notice her symptoms: "shortness of breath, cold sweat, fast heart, and very panicky." They indicate activation or damage to the nerves that initiate the *flight or fight reaction.* This is an acute stress reaction mediated by the autonomic nervous system, resulting in these same symptoms she suffered, shortness of breath, cold sweat, fast heartbeat, and panic. (The autonomic nervous system is a control system that acts largely unconsciously and regulates bodily functions such as the heart rate, digestion, respiratory rate, pupillary response, urination, and sexual arousal—*Wikipedia*)

I have mentioned repeatedly that the aging chemicals attack nerves. I suspect that many patients suffer from LCS and MSG with similarly severe and quick-acting fear reactions of the autonomic nervous system. The experience of this group of people suggests that many other people suffering similar symptoms react not to psychological instability but to MSG or MSG-like chemicals.

I have been stressing that food sensitivity is a slowly plodding beast that only starts after ingesting a quantity of dangerous food chemical that is more than the sensitive person can tolerate. Five sips of diet soda are hardly a large amount, and the resultant rapid attack is in no way slow. This quick reaction shows how—if a person is sensitive enough, in a reactive state, and eats or drinks a sensitizing chemical—the response can be far more rapid than expected.

Her symptoms indicate the power of the aging food chemicals—in this case, caused by LCSs—to irritate nerves and precipitate adverse reactions in body systems these nerves control, reactions such as headache pain.

Autonomic Nervous System Disorders: Dysautonomia

My patient's letter introduces us to disorders of the autonomic nervous system, also called *dysautonomia*. The Mayo Clinic defines it as nerve damage affecting involuntary bodily functions. With the information I provided and the information I will provide, I believe that you wonder, as I do, if the aging diet chemicals are the foremost causes of this autonomic nerve damage and a careful diet the best treatment.

Returning to my patient whose letter started us on this examination of the autonomic nervous system, I agree with her neighbor's pregnancy doctor: LCSs are poor choices during pregnancy.

6

Gluten

Gluten sensitivity is finally in the news. For years, I treated patients unaware they are gluten sensitive. After years of my wandering the grocery aisles looking for gluten-free foods and finding few, and after years of asking for a gluten-free menu at restaurants and encountering blank stares from servers, gluten is finally receiving the attention it deserves. Finally, many people know they suffer from gluten sensitivity; in stores, I find shelves of gluten-free foods; servers bring me the gluten-free menu I request. What a remarkable change—gluten is now not only famous but notorious.

What Is Gluten?

Gluten is a significant protein in the grains of the grass family (wheat, rye, barley, and oats). This protein is "sticky" and used in the baking industry to hold together bread, crackers, pastries, and other grain products. Because gluten has been in the news so often, you may be aware that many people believe they suffer health complications caused by gluten: You or a loved one may suffer from symptoms that you suspect are caused by gluten. If you do suspect it, there is a good chance you are right. In this chapter, I will increase your knowledge of gluten, its potential for causing harm to susceptible people, and how you can avoid this harm.

Many experts question whether *oat* gluten causes symptoms for gluten-sensitive people. I believe it does, although I confess that I am unsure it is. For now, I suggest that gluten-sensitive people avoid or reduce their consumption of foods made from oats. Corn also contains gluten, but not the same gluten as in the grass grains. Although many experts who treat celiac disease believe corn gluten is acceptable for their patients, I suspect—but cannot prove—that many patients sensitive to gluten also react to corn gluten, just not as severely. I hope to be able to examine these possibilities in the future.

My Discovery of Gluten

I do not criticize other doctors for failing to recognize that many patients suffer from gluten sensitivity. Even though I specialized in evaluating and treating patients suffering from food allergies and sensitivities—and have authored and published books on food allergies and sensitivities—I must admit that I was slow to recognize this common gluten sensitivity.

In my first book, published in 1991, *Treating Food Allergy, My Way,* I identified four aging chemicals: MSG, sugar, citric acid, and LCSs. But I had not yet recognized that lactose and gluten were also involved. Nor did I make a clear distinction between a food allergy and a food sensitivity.

In my book published in 1993, *Treating Sinus, Migraine and Cluster Headaches, My Way: An Allergist's Approach to Headache Treatment,* I described the importance of food allergies in causing headaches. However, I did not recognize the critical importance of food sensitivities but blamed "delayed food allergy."

It was only in my most recent book, published in 2000, *Food Allergies: The Complete Guide to Understanding and Relieving Your Food Allergies,* that I focused more heavily on the chemicals in foods—again discussing MSG, sugar, citric acid, and LCSs. Again, I underestimated the contribution of gluten to my patients' distress and did not indicate that gluten triggers sensitivity, not food allergy.

Food Allergy or Food Sensitivity

I am attempting to clarify the difference between food sensitivities and food allergies and discuss the sensitivity to the aging chemicals so common in our diet. I want to help you find and eat more helpful foods. I have already told you about the differences between a food allergy and a food sensitivity; now is an appropriate time to review these differences.

The Basic Cause

An overactive immune system causes food allergies and food sensitivity. This immune overreaction arises from the excessive consumption of the aging chemicals.

The Mediators of Harm

In food allergy, the immune system stimulates the release of quickly reacting antibodies that cause allergic symptoms such as hives, itching, swelling, wheezing, or abdominal distress. In food sensitivity, consuming more of the aging chemicals than we tolerate prompts a delayed immune reaction that irritates, damages, and ultimately destroys nerves resulting in many diseases of the body and mind.

Amounts Needed to Activate Symptoms

In a food allergy, a small amount of food can bring rapid-acting symptoms. More significant amounts are necessary to set off a reaction in food sensitivity: Symptoms typically appear only after excess consumption of these chemicals.

Difficulty in Diagnosis

A food allergy can usually be diagnosed by listening to patients' symptoms and is usually confirmed by skin and blood tests. Sensitivity to the aging chemicals is difficult to recognize by the patient's story and poorly diagnosed by tests. Test diets using reduced amounts of these chemicals or eliminating them from the diet help diagnose food sensitivity.

The Cause of Gluten Sensitivity

Briefly stated, gluten introduces excess MSG into the diet. Therefore, gluten sensitivity is also MSG sensitivity. Now you know why I needed to discuss MSG before putting gluten under our magnifying glass. I could have included gluten in the chapter on MSG but, because wheat, rye, barley, and oats are so important in our diet, gluten sensitivity deserves a chapter of its own.

Indications That MSG Causes Gluten Sensitivity

The strongest indications that MSG causes symptoms of gluten sensitivity are my patients' symptoms. Once I became aware of the surprising number of gluten-sensitive patients, I quickly learned that I could not diagnose my patients as gluten sensitive if they were not also sensitive to MSG. In many cases, my patients reacted to MSG some years before reacting to gluten. Without MSG sensitivity, I felt uncomfortable diagnosing gluten sensitivity.

The second indication that MSG is the cause of gluten sensitivity is the amount of glutamic acid in gluten. I discussed this already and will repeat it here because I believe this information is critical in understanding MSG sensitivity. This troubling amino acid, glutamic acid, is present and abundant in most proteins, usually forming about ten percent of the protein. In some proteins, including milk, corn, and soy, its levels are higher, about twenty percent. In wheat, the gluten level soars even more elevated.

When you consider the large amount of glutamic acid in gluten, it is easy to realize how it causes symptoms. This symptom promotion is especially understandable if the glutamic acid is loosely held in the gluten protein and escapes quickly from the protein when ingested and then rapidly absorbed. This rapid absorption in sensitive people overwhelms the weakened systems that prevent MSG's harm.

The third indication that MSG sensitivity and gluten sensitivity are the same is that they share the same symptoms. These symptoms are wide-ranging and include those below:

- Abdominal distention
- Abdominal distress
- Bloating
- Borborygmi (abdominal rumbling)
- Constipation

- Diarrhea
- Fatigue
- Headaches, migraines
- Hives
- Joint pains
- Nausea, vomiting
- Sweating, chills, clamminess, dizziness
- Weight loss

Symptoms Are Diverse

You may think: "This is not right. There are too many symptoms here; no medical condition can cause all of these symptoms. Aren't these people who claim they suffer from gluten sensitivity only imagining them?" The answer is no: These symptoms are all real and are caused by the aging chemicals, not by sufferers' imaginations.

What unites all these symptoms is that they have a single cause: injured nerves. The increased amounts of the neurostimulator, free glutamic acid, turns it into a neurotoxin, slowly poisoning the nerves controlling many critical systems of the body and brain, leading to multiple symptoms.

My patients suffered these various symptoms. I wondered why. For instance, Mary had migraine headaches, Jack suffered constipation, Kay and Jim felt very bloated, and Betty reacted with all of these symptoms. Why did Jack, Kay, and Jim not also suffer migraine headaches? I believe the answer lies in our genes. The Human Genome Project found in humans about 20,000 to 25,000 genes. Mary, Jack, Kay, Jim, and Betty have many gene differences that must make them susceptible to different symptoms.

The Human Genome Project also found that "switches" control the power of genes. Many genes have switches, and, over time, these switches slow, weaken, or dim the genes' actions—seriously hampering or weakening our control of MSG. The affected switches and genes can differ between people and cause the varying symptoms experienced by Mary, Jack, Kay, Jim, and Betty. So, the diversity of symptoms in gluten-sensitive people is not surprising but expected.

Why We Must Examine Celiac Disease Now

Celiac disease and sensitivity to the aging chemicals are similar because they both involve gluten. However, there are differences between these conditions, and these are essential differences. They permit food chemical-sensitive people to eat foods prohibited for celiac patients. The celiac diet is rigorous; the sensitivity diet is more relaxed. The diets must be different because the conditions are different, as I indicate below.

The Surface Lining of the Intestine

When celiac sufferers eat gluten, their immune systems attack the lining of their small intestines. The attack centers on the area of the intestine packed with tufts of hair-like strands called *villi*. Typically, food going through the intestine gets trapped, processed, and absorbed in these tufts. When celiac patients eat gluten, the immune system attacks these tufts, replacing them with a smooth surface like tile that does not allow food to cling to it, thereby slowing the absorption of food.

Sensitivity to the aging chemicals, on the other hand, does not attack the intestinal lining, so absorption of food continues without change.

Diagnosis by Lab Tests and Intestinal Biopsy
Doctors diagnose celiac disease by laboratory tests of the immune system and intestinal biopsy. Doctors cannot diagnose sensitivity to the aging chemicals by lab tests, intestinal biopsy, or x-ray.

Symptoms of Celiac Disease and Gluten Sensitivity
Celiac disease: As a result of the destruction of the villi, infants can suffer chronic diarrhea, swollen belly, pain, and failure to thrive. Older children are often overweight; some may suffer diarrhea, constipation, delayed puberty, or neurological symptoms. Adults usually display no digestive symptoms, although many have weight loss. Other symptoms include anemia, headaches, joint pain, heartburn, dental damage, and skin rash with blistering and itch.

Sensitivity to the aging chemicals: As already mentioned, symptoms occur in various systems due to damage to the nerves controlling those systems.

Consequences of Celiac Disease and
Sensitivity to the Aging Chemicals
The results of untreated celiac disease are damaging. These results include malnutrition, bone loss, infertility, and neurological symptoms, including numbness, tingling in the extremities, and balance loss. Untreated celiac disease patients also face an increased threat of certain cancers.

I detailed symptoms of sensitivity to the aging chemicals in the list above. In general, their symptoms are pain and discomfort and not the more severe symptoms accompanying celiac disease in adults. Prolonged damage to and destruction of nerves in this disorder due to the aging chemicals may have tragic consequences, including deterioration of the brain's nerves.

Lactose Sensitivity

I will discuss lactose sensitivity in Chapter 9.

In celiac disease, lactose sensitivity occurs due to impaired digestion because of damage to the villi.

Treatment of Celiac Disease and Gluten Sensitivity

Treatment of celiac disease is complete gluten avoidance.

Treatment of sensitivity to the aging chemicals: Treatment consists of lowering the consumption of the troubling chemicals to an amount tolerated by the individual.

Summary

Sensitivity to these chemicals that promote aging is caused by ingesting more of them than we can tolerate. Diagnosis by laboratory tests or biopsy is difficult; therefore, no long-term peer-reviewed studies can tell us the eventual consequences of this sensitivity except for the already-known damaging effects the chemicals have on the nervous system. Now that we have examined gluten, LCSs, and MSG, it is time to tell you about another troublesome food chemical, an essential chemical: refined sugar.

7
Refined Sugar

What Is Refined Sugar?

Refined sugar belongs to the carbohydrate class of chemicals and comprises just three elements: carbon, hydrogen, and oxygen. Monosaccharides (mono—one, saccharide—sugar) are the carbohydrates class to which glucose and fructose belong. They are simple sugars. When chemically united, they make the disaccharide (di—two, saccharides—sugar) sucrose.

Sucrose is the sugar you spoon into your coffee, mix with flour to make sweet treats, and that you find in many processed foods. It comes mainly from three sources: beet sugar from sugar beets, cane sugar from sugar cane, and corn sugar, often called high-fructose corn syrup, from corn. Glucose, fructose, and sucrose are all simple sugars.

Since the chemical compositions of the sucrose in cane and beet sugar are similar, we will treat them as identical. High-fructose corn sugar has other carbohydrates in addition to sucrose, and we will treat this sugar with care.

Molasses, honey, fruit nectars, maple syrup, cane juice, and agave nectar are sugars—food manufacturers add them to processed foods to sweeten the foods. On food and beverage labels, terms like "added sugars" signal their presence.

Sugars Found in Foods

In many foods naturally rich in sugar, such as potatoes, the sugar is composed mainly of glucose bound together as starch. Potatoes also contain fructose. Boiling the potatoes lowers the content of fructose because some of this sugar dissolves into the boiling water. The amount of fructose in bread depends on the amount of sucrose added as the dough is formed. Many fruits naturally contain elevated levels of fructose, including grapes, apples, bananas, kiwi fruit, mangos, sweet cherries, pears, and pineapples. Juices made from fruits contain the sugars of these fruits and add these sugars to the diet when ingested.

Now let's turn our attention to why we worry so much about refined sugar. The refined sugars in our diet play the role of a villain: I worry about these villainous tendencies. Sugar harms us because of a mistake in logic made by many people—including my fellow medical doctors. Many doctors blamed the wrong foods in their well-meaning fight against their patients' obesity, diabetes, and other diseases. In the past, they blamed fatty foods such as eggs, beef, and pork for causing obesity and heart disease while failing to implicate one of the real culprits: refined sugars. Many of today's medical researchers are reexamining these thoughts. They actively seek out sugar's role in causing many common conditions.

My Experience With Refined Sugar

To help you understand how I feel about sugar, let me tell you about my own experience with it. I am a typical sufferer from the aging chemicals, and I use what I learned from my experiences with these chemicals to help you understand the harm they cause. The people susceptible to the damage the aging chemicals cause the body and brain—and who continue to eat our modern diet—can suffer the same harm sugar caused me (and still would trouble me if I do not follow my diet). Through my writing and speaking, I try to lead sugar-sensitive people away from foods with excess sugar and guide them toward eating a diet that will reverse some of the harm sugar causes.

I reacted to sugar: I was obese. At one time, I was five feet eight inches tall and weighed 250 pounds. Heavy? My suits were extra-large.

I knew I had to lose weight, but I knew I lacked the will-power to follow a strict weight-loss diet; I had to find another way to rid myself of fat. I decided that I could tolerate changing one aspect of my diet—I could eliminate sweet treats. So, I did. I ate as much unsweetened food as I wanted, as often as I wanted. I lost about five to ten pounds a year, year after year until my weight dropped from 248 pounds to 200 pounds. I was pleased.

Then, some years later, after I had identified the other aging food chemicals, I changed my diet to decrease the amount of these other foods in my diet. Slowly, my weight lessened further as I lost a further fifty pounds. Altogether, just through these diet changes, I lost 100 pounds!

While I carried this extra weight, I also experienced bloating. As my weight dropped, my bloated subsided. My patients following the diet also lost their bloating as they lost weight.

Surprising Remarks by Two Patients

Two patients suffering headaches startled me with their comments. Both were following my diet guidelines, and both returned to my office in the same week. Both mentioned that the diet relieved their headaches. They also told me how much better they felt as their bloating and abdominal distress subsided. Then, they both said, "And I lost thirty pounds!" From their expressions, I could tell that this weight loss startled them as much as the coincidence of their comments surprised me. Their experience of feeling less bloated and losing weight coincided precisely with mine. This coincidence of two people losing the same amount of weight, telling me about it in the same words—and in the same week—brought the relationship between bloating and diet forcibly to my attention.

Studies on Refined Sugar

Current diet research agrees with my experiences: You can expect to lose weight if you avoid the food chemicals that cause aging, especially refined sugar.

Gary Taubes described studies on sugar, and what he discovered can be found in his book, *Why We Get Fat: and What to Do About It*. Taubes has spent years of journalistic research on diet and chronic diseases, and I believe he writes with great authority. In his article for the *New York Times* magazine titled "Is Sugar Toxic?" (April 13, 2011), he discusses the evidence for this toxicity as he reviews research by Dr. Robert Lustig.

Dr. Lustig was a pediatric obesity specialist and treated many obese children at his clinic at the University of California, San Francisco. On May 26, 2009, he discussed sugar in a lecture titled "Sugar: The Bitter Truth." His talks were popular, and millions visited his website. Because he studied these issues and treated obese patients, he had theoretical knowledge of obesity through his research and teaching and a practical understanding of obesity through his patient care. In short, he was an expert, and his thoughts are still pertinent today.

In his discussion of refined sugar, Dr. Lustig called it a *poison* and a *toxin*. I also believe that sugar is toxic or poisonous to people sensitive to the aging chemicals and who eat and drink sugar-flavored treats above their tolerance. He thought they suffer toxicity leading to diseases. I agree. He described studies that show that our modern diet leads to this excess, pointing out that:

- Excess refined sugar causes disease.
- Nobody chooses to suffer illness.
- Glucose does not cause this disease.
- Fructose, consumed in excess, causes disease.
- Excess fructose weakens the hormone signal that we have eaten enough food.
- Avoiding excess fructose reduces the threat of illness.
- Eating less food does not eliminate fructose's threat.
- Exercise improves muscle tone, health, and mental ability.

Excess Refined Sugar Causes Disease

In his *New York Times* magazine article, Gary Taubes points out that the U.S. Department of Agriculture estimated that in 1980 Americans were eating and drinking seventy-five pounds of refined sugar per person each year. By early 2000, we had increased our yearly intake of refined sugar to ninety pounds. With this rising consumption, more of us became obese.

In 1980, one in seven Americans suffered from obesity, while in early 2000, one in three Americans suffered from obesity. The United States went from six million diabetics in 1980 to fourteen million diabetics in 2000. Although other factors encourage the emergence of obesity and diabetes, this parallel rise in sugar intake, obesity, and diabetes significantly points to sugar as a major cause.

Nobody Chooses to Suffer Diseases

Most people agree with this thought. Our diet causes many diseases, but here I will discuss the obesity caused by our diet. Obese people regret their obesity. Carrying excess weight is tiring, uncomfortable, and unhealthy. Other children bully overweight children, overweight adolescents have difficulty dating, and overweight adults face distressing choices in clothing. Overweight people are also at increased risk of low self-esteem.

Nobody chooses to be overweight. Unfortunately, many are stuck with obesity until they understand why they are obese and learn to live and eat in such a way that the pounds drop away. I believe this is true of most people suffering from obesity, but I also realize that people who, because of genetic makeup or mental or physical illness, cannot lose their extra pounds. They should not be condemned but should be evaluated and treated by specialists in obesity. As for people suffering the many diseases caused by our diet, none of them chose these illnesses. Knowing the dietary causes of these illnesses will help them fight this excess fat.

Glucose Does not Cause Disease

It is not the sugar called glucose that causes diet-related disease. Fruits and vegetables contain glucose, and our bodies have significant stores of it. Glucose provides the primary source of our body's energy, and every cell of our body uses it. When we eat glucose-containing foods, most of the sugar travels to the cells throughout our bodies, enters these cells, and uses the glucose. Some glucose becomes stored in the liver in glycogen that is readily converted into glucose to produce energy—a process harmless for the body.

Fructose Causes Disease

When we eat or drink the various foods and beverages sweetened with refined sugar, as in sucrose and high-fructose corn syrup, their fructose and glucose contents quickly enter the body.

In contrast to glucose that every cell in the body can absorb and use, fructose is mainly shunted into the liver because only the liver can metabolize it. In mammals like us, the liver turns much of excess fructose into fat and, at the same time, releases insulin from the pancreas in significant amounts. This oversupply of insulin reaches a stage where we can no longer maintain this increased insulin release and become insulin resistant or diabetic. This process helps explain diabetes in humans.

Along with this insulin resistance comes increased triglycerides, a fat that helps narrow arterial blood vessels, a pathway through which humans suffer heart attacks and strokes.

The question arises: If fructose is so dangerous, why are we using it? The answers are multiple: We thought the fat in our diet, not sugar, was causing heart disease and strokes; high fructose corn syrup is cheap and plentiful; fructose is sweet, almost twice as sweet as glucose, and we need it to make our sweet treats sweet. We did not recognize its danger.

Excess Fructose Weakens the Hormone Signal That We Have Eaten Enough Food

In addition to causing diabetes, insulin resistance induced by excess fructose ingestion seriously increases the sensation of hunger and retards feeling full. Three hormones control how we react to foods: Ghrelin signals the brain that the body is hungry, leptin signals that appetite is satisfied, and insulin reinforces the signal that the body has eaten enough. When we become resistant to insulin, the indication that we are full becomes less effective, causing insulin-resistant people to feel great hunger despite eating sufficient food. They then overeat and become obese. Combining constant hunger and overindulgence in sweet foods and beverages with body fat resulting from consuming fructose leads to obesity.

Avoiding Excess Fructose Reduces the Threat of Disease

I believe this point is clear. Avoiding or eliminating the foods and drinks with excess fructose fights obesity and other diseases associated with the fructose of refined sugar. Removing the foods that degrade the satiety signaling (the signal which says that you are full) means that after a meal, the stomach feels pleasantly full, reducing the tendency to overeat and promoting weight loss. Unless there is some complicating medical or psychological complication, people avoiding fructose should lose weight.

Eating Less Food Does Not Eliminate Fructose's Threat

Obese people can lose weight by starving themselves, but they are not attacking the root causes of their obesity. The aging chemicals are root causes. As long as the obese eat and drink more aging chemicals than they tolerate, insulin and leptin signaling weakens, they remain hungry and do not enjoy the sensation of feeling full. Obese people suffer continual hunger, and any lost weight quickly returns.

Exercise Improves Muscle Tone, Health, and Mental Ability

Exercise is essential for your health. If you use refined sugar to excess, it will be hard for you to perform enough activity to rid yourself of excess weight. You will carry this added fat while you exercise, making the exercise exhausting.

To lose this added fat despite eating and drinking the aging chemicals, you will need to exercise like a committed athlete, performing hours of moderate-to high-intensity exercise. It takes hours of intense exercise to shed an appreciable amount of fat. If your workout is less severe and prolonged, the fat derived from your consumed fructose will remain.

However, if you are a committed athlete, you should already know that you need glucose-based glycogen, not fructose-based fat, for energy storage and use during exercise. Both glucose and its storage form, glycogen, rapidly release energy during periods of activity. Glucose acts like gasoline that activates your car's motor; it rapidly changes to energy. That's why many athletes load up on glucose—not refined sugar—when they are doing carbohydrate loading.

Further, if you continue to eat processed sugar, with exercise you will still suffer hunger despite eating meals that should satisfy your need. If you succumb to the temptation to eat food and drink beverages with excess refined sugar, you will add more fat to your overburdened body.

These factors help explain why exercise, by itself, does not counteract obesity. However, exercise and changing your diet, significantly lowering the amount of fructose-containing refined sugar, counteract obesity. By avoiding fructose, you can eat more energy-yielding glucose, add it to your energy stores as glycogen, and reactivate the satiety hormones. You should also feel far healthier and younger.

My Experience With Avoiding Excess Refined Sugar

My experience agrees with the above. As long as I avoid sweet treats, I can eat three meals a day and many snacks between meals and still lose weight. I feel content and do not want any food for hours. I do not miss sweet treats. (Unless I eat even one bite. Then I want more! That is sugar addiction!)

Additionally, in the past, my blood pressure was elevated. After avoiding excess refined sugar, my blood pressure is lower, and I do not take medicine to lower my blood pressure.

Current research on carbohydrates predicts these results; if you avoid fructose, you have a great chance of experiencing the same results.

Where to Find Refined Sugar

Look for sugar on the list of ingredients printed on the labels of foods (this may not be a complete list):

- Any sugar (cane, corn, beet sugar)
- Any juice
- Any syrup (corn syrup, maple syrup)
- Agave
- Barley malt
- Caramel
- Dextrose
- Diastatic malt
- Fructose
- Galactose
- Glucose or glucose solids
- Golden syrup
- Honey
- Jaggery
- Lactose
- Maltodextrin
- Maltose
- Molasses
- Panela
- Panoche
- Rapadura
- Sucanat
- Sucrose
- Treacle

As I mentioned, our fruits contain significant amounts of fructose. Fruits, including apple, pear, and berries, are extensively modified from the original, natural fruits by selecting for enlarged size and increased sweetness.

Our Diet Causes Many Diseases

The role of sugar in obesity, diabetes and dementia is well studied, but they are not the only diseases caused by our diet. Sugar is one of the aging chemicals in our diet and, in excess, acts as a whole-body poison and contributes to diseases of mind and body. As the list of conditions is long, I use obesity and diabetes as examples of these diseases, but I acknowledge the other diseases caused by our diet. Disorders of the mind, including depression, also improve with the Mediterranean diet, which avoids sugar. Because of experiences with children, the relationship of sugar with hyperactivity fascinates me.

Hyperactivity

Now let's examine how sugar causes hyperactivity.

Unfortunately, researchers have difficulty agreeing that sugar causes hyperactivity. The doubters do not believe it does. Some studies agree, studies that drew their conclusions by contrasting the behavior of two groups of children with one group eating a diet with sucrose (table sugar) and another group an LCS. The researchers noticed no difference in the activities of the two groups.

These studies prove that sugar does not cause hyperactivity, or they prove that children suffer similar hyperactivity from refined sugar and LCSs. I think the latter interpretation is correct.

Nerve stimulation and irritation are reasonable explanations for the hyperactivity of children following sweet treats. A very wise elementary school teacher I know, Kevin, once remarked (and I paraphrase): "Thank goodness that this year there was no school the day after Halloween. With all that candy, the kids are uncontrollable!"

When my grandchildren were younger, and I cared for them overnight, I learned to bargain with them. They can have a sugary treat, but they must go to bed on time if they do. Without that bargain, I found it hard to slow them down enough to get them to bed.

These two examples are, to me, sufficient proof that sugar causes hyperactivity. When we accept the proposition that hyperactivity is caused or worsened by a central nervous system toxic effect, it enhances the possibility that refined sugar hyper-excites nerves. Further strengthening this possibility are studies that show that reducing sugar intake quiets many disorders of the mind.

I believe the information I presented in this chapter suggests that it is wise to avoid refined sugar in the quest to fight against diseases of mind and body. It suggests that this hyperactivity of fructose damages the brain's nerves in those susceptible to dementia.

8

Citrus Acids

Citrus acids include citric, malic, fumaric, succinic, and tartaric acid. I classify these acids as citrus acids because they have the same potential for harm as citric acid.

I served in the United States Air Force after completing my medical internship and before my allergy/immunology residency. I was unsure of which field of medicine I would join: I knew I might specialize in allergy treatment as this specialty attracted me because of my allergies. With these thoughts and with the consent of our commander, I started the allergy clinic at the air force base.

One of my patients, a little girl about ten years old, Joyce, taught me much (none of the names used in the following story are actual names). She suffered from a severe rash called eczema or atopic dermatitis. Unfortunately, my treatment was giving her little relief. Her skin was as red and raw as if it was scraped with sandpaper. I pitied her.

Joyce's Story

One day, her father brought her to my office, and her skin was as soft and unmarked as a baby's skin. I said, "Well, finally, my treatment worked. I am so glad!"

He replied, "Doctor Walsh, my wife and I appreciate your efforts to help our little girl, but your treatment gave her little relief."

With my pride profoundly punished, I asked her father, "Well, why is her skin so clear?"

He replied, "Because she treats herself! When her skin breaks out, she draws her bathwater, pours kitchen cleanser into it, sits in it, and washes. Her bath ends her itch, and her skin clears." I was shocked at this improbable story, but I had to believe her father. After all of medicine's conventional eczema treatments failed, her kitchen cleanser bath gave her great relief.

She Treated Her Eczema

Although my experience with Joyce taught me something new about eczema—something absent from my medical training—I did not know what it was teaching me. Was I supposed to tell my eczema patients to wash with kitchen cleanser? I really couldn't because that would not be conventional treatment, and therefore, it was too much like medical experimentation, and I would not subject my patients to experiments. Although I suspected that the cleanser treatment caused no harm, I was not sure whether it was safe.

Even though I didn't know what her story was trying to teach me, I never forgot it. Like a jigsaw puzzle with a vital piece missing, this missing puzzle piece might teach me more about eczema than all my medical books. It could teach me how to treat this miserably itchy skin rash.

Craig's Story: The Missing Puzzle Piece

I found that missing puzzle piece years later while practicing as an allergy/immunologist specialist after finishing my allergy fellowship at the Mayo Clinic. A boy and his mother supplied it. It was—to me—information so radical, so stunning, and so valuable that it unlocked the secret to treating many cases of eczema.

I liked his mother; she was an intelligent and honest person and a great mother to her son, Craig. Like Joyce, Craig was a child with severe eczema. His skin, also like Joyce's, was red and raw and extremely itchy.

I still can picture Craig's mother in my mind and remember our conversation, and it went like this: "Mary, our treatment does not help Craig, does it?"

"No, it doesn't."

Still looking for that piece of the jigsaw puzzle, I asked her, "Do you have any feeling for what is causing his skin rash?"

She replied, "Yes, he breaks out from citric acid."

What the Stories Taught Me

Wow! Impossible! My medical school professors never told me that citric acid causes eczema. Mary and I agreed that she would take away all the citrus from Craig's diet to see if her incredible observation was accurate—that citric acid caused his eczema. She came back to see me with Craig in two weeks. Incredibly, his skin was much clearer, perhaps a fifty percent improvement. She was right—that improvement meant that citric acid was a cause of his eczema.

However, the remaining fifty percent bothered me, and I questioned Mary about any other causes she might have noticed, but unfortunately, she knew of no other reason.

I thought about Mary's observation about citrus, realizing it might be a piece of the jigsaw puzzle I was seeking.

Combining Craig's story with what Joyce had taught me about her kitchen-cleanser bath, I could think of one connection between these two events: Sensitivity to citric acid causes eczema! When Joyce or Craig ate or drank too much citrus, their bodies excreted the excess citrus onto the skin, irritating the nerves of their skin as the acid passed through the skin, causing the skin to itch. The itching caused the eczema rash. Therefore, eczema rash is an acid burn of the skin.

That explained why Joyce's skin healed with the kitchen-cleanser bath. The alkaline cleanser neutralized the citric acid and then washed it away, allowing the skin to heal. None of the recommended eczema treatments I used matched the effectiveness of the cleanser. This experience alerted me to a monstrous problem: Allergists were unaware that citric acid made millions of miserable people itch and scratch. Further, if we were unaware of this food chemical sensitivity to acids, how many other troubling food sensitivities lurked undiagnosed in our patients?

I knew that there must be other food chemicals involved in the rash because Craig's skin, although improved by eliminating citrus, was still troubled. I suspected that the mysterious something was in his diet—another troublesome food chemical like citric acid that I had not identified.

This thought increased my search for the other food chemicals, and I found the food chemicals that age us and cause my patients' severe skin itch. Among these discoveries was that other acids caused the same distress as citric acid, the acids of the citrus acid group (see below).

I wish I had known about these chemicals when I was

treating Craig. I would have immediately suspected sugar, MSG, and other citrus acids. I was also unaware of the many foods and beverages flavored by these acids. I believe Craig's skin rash would have relented, and his torment subsided further if I had that information at that time.

Telling you the stories of these children allows me to discuss several concepts including sensitivity to citric acid, the skin condition called eczema, and eczema treatment.

Citrus Acids

Malic, tartaric, fumaric, and succinic acids have similarities with citric acid, and we will look at them here.

Citric Acid

Citric acid is a natural, weak organic acid found in many fruits and vegetables, especially citrus fruits. Our bodies naturally contain citric acid and use it for several purposes, including producing the body's energy through the citric acid cycle. The body tolerates this natural content of citric acid. However, when citrus-sensitive people consume excess citric acid, they react.

The excessive amounts of citric acid in the modern diet are new; citric acid was relatively recently isolated, identified, and brought to the diet. It has not been a part of our diet long enough for us to be genetically programmed to handle it. To restate this: In people sensitive to citric acid, the genes and the switches that control these genes have not had the many thousands of years necessary to acquire the gene modifications allowing us to handle the amount of citrus acids we consume.

Malic Acid

Like citric acid, malic acid is in the cells of our bodies and present in the foods we eat. Also, like citric acid, it participates in the citric acid energy cycle. Unlike the glutamic acid in MSG with no taste of its own, malic acid brings out a robust, fruity flavor in food and beverages. While citric acid gives foods and drinks a pronounced sour taste, malic acid's contribution is a milder sourness persisting longer than the taste of citric acid.

The amount of malic acid produced and used in the body is not a danger; it can handle the acids it makes and uses daily. And we can ignore the usual dietary levels of malic acid in foods since the amount in the foods and beverages is typically low, and sensitive people tolerate the small amount of this acid just as they tolerate limited amounts of the other aging food chemicals. Only when a person's diet includes excess amounts of the food chemicals like citric or malic acid will the body suffer.

I was never able, through questioning my patients, to gauge the degree of harm caused by malic acid. Once they learned that food chemicals caused their symptoms, they stopped eating and drinking excessive amounts of candies, gum, desserts, bakery products, and other processed foods and diet soft drinks that contain malic acid flavoring. The few who returned to eating and drinking these foods and beverages suffered symptoms like painful headaches, annoying sleeplessness, or cramping abdominal pain, reinforcing their commitment to avoiding these troubling food chemicals.

Fumaric Acid

The story is the same with fumaric acid, which is the sourest of the food acids; the amount produced and used daily the body handles well. I believe it possesses the same nerve-injury power as citric and glutamic acid. Still, fewer people suffer from sensitivity because there is far less of it in the diet for sensitive people to eat and drink.

Succinic Acid

Succinic acid is another relative of this group of acids. It seems to be growing in popularity as its synthesis becomes easier. My patients had limited exposure to it.

Tartaric Acid

Tartaric acid is an acid not found in large quantities in the body but found in many plants, especially grapes—and in the wine made from grapes. Wine makes some people feel sick, and its content of tartaric acid may be a reason for this distress (the roof of my mouth swelled with eating grapes). Sensitive people should limit their consumption of wine if they tolerate tartaric acid poorly.

Diseases From Excess Amounts of Citrus Acids

Eczema/Atopic Dermatitis

"Eczema" is a nonspecific term for many types of skin inflammation. The eczema we are discussing is atopic dermatitis is a long-lasting, chronic skin rash that causes intense skin itching. The term atopic comes from "atopy," which means "associated with or caused by an allergy." In some eczema sufferers, a food or inhalant allergy aggravates the rash. Further suggesting allergy, other allergic symptoms such as hay fever and allergic asthma often accompany atopic dermatitis. However, in my allergy practice, sensitivity to excess citrus acids was a more potent cause of the rash than a true allergy.

In infancy, eczema or atopic dermatitis appears mainly on the face and scalp (probably from a combination of the citric acid found in mother's milk and from the mechanical rubbing of the face against the sheets) and often in the diaper area, most likely from the citric acid in the stool and urine. The associated rash can be so severe it causes blisters that ooze and crust over. An estimated one in five babies suffers from this rash, so it is a common condition. In adults, the rash appears as red to off-red patches that at times have small, raised bumps that leak fluid—in severe cases, as with Joyce and Craig—scratching brings a crusty, itching rawness to the skin.

The rash from eczema can appear all over the body, or it can be most severe at the ankles and wrists. Characteristic sites of involvement are at the bends of the elbow and behind the knees (this may be because these areas have softer, more irritation-prone skin that perspires more—lending credibility to the theory of citrus acids excreted from the body through sweat). It also occurs on the hands, resulting in dishwasher's hands (a combination of dryness of the hands from sensitivity to citrus acids and washing clothes and dishes).

Eczema rash differs from the rash of contact dermatitis, which can also be red, raw, and itchy. Contact dermatitis usually begins with tiny fluid-filled swellings of the skin appearing quickly (in minutes) or slowly (hours) after touching whatever chemical is causing the contact dermatitis. Severe contact dermatitis irritates, itches, and hurts much more than the itch from severe atopic dermatitis. (For reference, a common cause of contact dermatitis is the oil from the poison ivy plant.)

The Acid Regulatory System

A possible cause of eczema, a cause that I believe is the leading cause, is that citrus acids are poisonous when consumed in excess, and the body tries to rid itself of these acids in any way possible. Many people can eliminate these acids by flushing them out through sweat or tears. The acids in these watery discharges burn the skin around the eyes (that happens to me) or on other areas of the body, subject to acid sweating, leading to the burning itch of eczema.

Eczema/Atopic Dermatitis in Infants and Adults

Eczema in Infants and Children

Many people suffer from eczema; it is a significant problem. It affects many infants and young children. As they are not aged, their ability to tolerate citrus acids should not have been weakened because of their age.

I believe the best explanation for this sensitivity in the young is that the body does not want to tolerate excesses of these acids, no matter its age. Some babies will have the ability to discharge these acids even as infants. In some rare cases of atopic dermatitis, genes that predispose to the rash have been identified. Whatever the cause, treatment includes:

- Reducing the amount of citrus acids in the breastfeeding mother's diet.

- Reducing citrus acids in the formula fed to the infant.
- Avoid providing the acids to the young child.

These measures may significantly relieve the rash, and the citrus acids can be returned to the diet if the avoidance does not improve the skin.

Eczema in Adults

That citric acid sensitivity affects adults is no surprise as older people lose their ability to tolerate the excess citrus acids just like they suffer weakening of their ability to handle extra sugar and MSG. In adults, the treatment that limits the excess citrus acids in the diet often brings welcome relief.

Current Treatment and Prevention of Eczema

Current eczema treatment includes using a mild soap to avoid drying out the skin and a moisturizer to conserve the body's natural moisture immediately after a bath. For years, doctors treating adults suffering from eczema have told them to take warm, short showers (because hot, long showers dry out the skin) and reduce any stress that may worsen the itchiness. Doctors suggested using medicines such as over-the-counter topical hydrocortisone and antihistamines for mild eczema. They often treated adult sufferers of severe eczema with oral cortisone, ultraviolet light treatment, immunosuppressant/immunomodulatory drugs, and prescription-strength cortisone lotions.

The following measures are suggested: lightly patting the skin dry within three minutes of bathing or showering; using moisturizers daily; using a humidifier; wearing soft clothing;

avoiding temperature changes and sweating; keeping finger-nails short to reduce the harm caused by scratching and even removing carpeting from living spaces and treating pets for dander.

The treatment Joyce and Craig taught me, including re-ducing the amount of citrus acids in the diet, may be more successful than all these suggestions, if it is tried. Sometimes, out of frustration, I yearn to shake those treating patients with eczema and say, "Instead of all these actions to relieve and prevent the itch, tell your patients to reduce the amount of acids reaching their skin. Try citrus acid avoidance; it's safe, and it should relieve many of your suffering eczema patients!"

Other Symptoms of Sensitivity to Citrus Acids

Cold Sores/Fever Blisters

One peculiar but widespread symptom of citric acid sensitiv-ity is cold sores or fever blisters. They are small but annoying fluid-filled blisters, usually around the lips and in the mouth that break easily, discharging their watery fluid and then forming a crust as they heal. The nerves supplying these un-comfortable skin sections are not protecting the skin. Citrus acids do not initiate these cold sores; blame the sores on a virus that quietly infects the nerves that control and protect the lips and mouth. Activation of this virus in the nerves by another virus, for instance a cold virus, so injures nerves that they can no longer protect the area that they should con-trol, allowing the involved area to progress into a cold sore. In many citrus-sensitive people, I discovered that eating or drinking citrus acids powerfully irritate and worsen these virus-damaged nerves, pointing out that they share the power of sugar and MSG to damage nerves.

Eating and drinking more citric acid than a person tolerates worsens the distress of the cold sores, including how frequently they appear, their size, the discomfort they cause, their duration and their unsightliness. It also increases the number of cold sores that erupt with each episode. I know this is so because these complications affect many of my patients and also affect me.

If I avoid foods and beverages with excess citrus acids, any cold sores that develop will remain small and unnoticed. If I have too much of the citrus acids, one or more large, very noticeable and annoying cold sores grow on my lips or the roof of my mouth.

I remember very well a patient who suffered many years of cold sores, each involving a crop of sores numbering up to fourteen, appearing in many areas all over his mouth and lips. He was shocked to hear that citric acid may make the cold sores so miserable—and equally shocked when avoiding citrus dramatically reduced these miserable sores.

A Teachable Moment: A Mouth Swelling

One other event helped me understand the potency of citrus acids in injuring nerves. I had convinced myself that I could tolerate the amount of acid in table grapes and ate them every morning for breakfast. After several weeks of indulging in these little taste balls, the entire roof of my mouth swelled up. I realized the most likely explanation for the swelling was that the citrus and tartaric acids in the grapes damaged the nerves that maintained the integrity of the roof of my mouth.

These nerves were not able to continue protecting it, and it swelled. I immediately stopped eating grapes; the swelling lasted three weeks and then subsided, leaving no lasting damage. The episode left me with a good lesson in the ability of the citrus acid to irritate and damage nerves.

This episode, although uncomfortable, led me to the following conclusions: As a known sufferer from the effects of the aging chemicals, I cannot tolerate excess acid from grapes. As it is a sensitivity and not an allergy, I can still eat grapes but only in amounts that do not stress my tolerance. Actually, after that experience, I will not eat them. The episode reinforced the concept that citrus acids in excess are nerve toxins. My recovery again showed me that nerves can return to normal function by avoiding the food that damaged them. This recovery of the function of nerves is an important concept: Damaged Nerves Can Recover! That is, as long as the sufferer does not wait too long to change the diet.

Finding Citrus Acids

Citrus fruits and juice have the highest natural concentrations of the citrus acids—oranges, lemons, limes, and grapefruit—with lemons containing the most citric acid in this group. Other fruits containing appreciable amounts of the acids include apple, apricot, cherry, grapefruit, grapes, mango, peach, pear, pineapple, strawberry, and watermelon. I limit my intake of fruits and juices. I could exceed my tolerance by drinking citrus-flavored drinks, which are identified by their fruity taste and by reading the list of ingredients: I no longer drink them. Citrus acids known for adding "brightness" to many food flavors are used in Mediterranean and Far Eastern dishes and flavor many fish dishes. I am uncomfortable with the inclusion of these acids in my diet or the diet of others with dementia or other diet-caused diseases.

Summary

I fear excess consumption of these food acids. I believe they have great potential for harm. In many of my patients, citrus acids show their potential for significant damage by causing or worsening many cases of atopic dermatitis and cold sores.

We know that chronic indolent virus infection of the facial nerves causes cold sores, and I found that these acids significantly worsen these cold sores. Various studies also show that the chickenpox virus, herpes zoster, quietly infects the body's nerves. Reactivation of this virus causes the severely itchy/painful skin rash called shingles, which typically appears on the face or body and is most likely worsened by the citric acid we eat and drink.

Studies indicate that herpes and other viruses can also invade and chronically infect the brain's nerves. This chronic brain infection may worsen with the consumption of excess citrus acids. I believe these acids injure brain tissue as they injure the body's nerves in cold sores, shingles, atopic dermatitis, and the swelling of the mouth I experienced. If consuming excess citric acid stops in time, nerves in the brain and body can recover. However, if excess consumption of citric acid continues in people with chronic nerve damage, this damage may become permanent, and they can lose nerve-dependent abilities permanently.

People sensitive to citrus acids do not need to avoid these food acids strictly. Prevention or recovery from nerve damage may just entail limiting the amount consumed to the amount tolerated.

In this chapter and previous chapters, I told you about some characteristics of the food chemicals that age us. I described how each chemical injures nerves. Citrus acids belong in this group; some of the damage caused by excess intake is readily apparent: rashes, mouth swelling, and cold sores. Some damage may hide from you, but that does not make them less destructive. I fear these acids are significant causes of damage to the central nervous system in the dementias. People fearing the onset, or suffering from, these diseases should look carefully at their diets.

9

Lactose (Milk Sugar)

Lactose is a sugar in human and cow's milk. For our discussion of the aging chemicals, lactose is helpful because we can apply studies of milk to the other aging chemicals. Scientists are aware of why people react to it, and researchers pursued creditable peer-reviewed clinical studies of this sensitivity. Doctors now have evidence-based methods of treatment. However, despite this increased knowledge, the role lactose plays in nerve injury and destruction is not as straightforward as the role of the other food chemicals.

The Aging Food Chemicals Must Include Lactose

Lactose still must be included in this discussion because, in my many patients suffering from these aging chemicals, lactose sensitivity was almost always present. If patients denied sensitivity to lactose and offered convincing proof they were not sensitive, such as drinking more than one glass of cow's milk each day without exhibiting symptoms, I doubted that they suffered from the aging chemicals. But, almost always, they failed to provide this proof. I cannot remember a food chemical-sensitive patient who was not also sensitive to lactose. Lactose joins the other chemicals as either a cause of nerve damage or an "innocent bystander" linked to them like each link of a chain connects to the next.

My lactose-sensitive patients who told me that they were not sensitive were not lying when they denied their sensitivity: They thought I was asking about milk *allergy*. They did not realize that lactose sensitivity is not an allergy; with milk *allergy*, even a small amount of milk causes quickly appearing hives, tongue swelling, or other uncomfortable and sometimes dangerous symptoms. Food *sensitivity* usually arises slowly—even sluggishly—hours after a meal when the sensitive person eats or drinks more of the specific food or beverage than she can tolerate.

When my patients denied being lactose sensitive, I became anxious that I was considering the wrong diagnosis. My anxiety would usually evaporate when I asked: "How much milk do you drink in a day?" When they answered, "Only enough for cereal in the morning," I knew my patients had limited tolerance for lactose, making it more likely they had limited toleration to the other aging chemicals. This toleration was usually four ounces of lactose-containing milk each day. If they told me that they drank more than four ounces, I asked if they suffered from intestinal gas. If they answered "yes," I knew the cause of the gas was lactose, and I could be comfortable with the diagnosis of milk and food chemical sensitivity. If they answered "no," I became very uncomfortable with my diagnosis and started looking for another diagnosis.

Patients Deny the Cause of Their Illness

As a doctor, I found that typically patients are intelligent and observant, possessing great *street smarts*. Subconsciously, most of them knew—before they came to me for evaluation—the foods that caused their discomfort. However, because they enjoyed these foods, they had trouble admitting their sensitivity to themselves.

I learned that my task was to elevate awareness of their sensitivity from their subconscious minds, where it lay hidden, to their conscious minds, where they could acknowledge their sensitivity and deal with it. I could see in their faces the struggle to avoid accepting my diagnosis. I needed sympathy and kindness to help them achieve their acceptance. If my diagnosis was correct, I could follow the play of emotion across their faces that transitioned from "No! That cannot be right!" to "OMG, it is right!" Then came the smile that said, "All right, I have been hiding it from myself." These words, although apparent in their facial expressions, were seldom spoken to me.

Some patients, however, could not admit—even to themselves—that the foods they craved made them suffer. They told me flat-out, "I cannot accept that diagnosis." I thanked them for their honesty, wished I had the tests to tell them that my diagnosis was correct, and hoped they would have good luck finding another diagnosis and treatment that would give them relief. Typically, I could not refer them to another doctor because their primary doctor—and then perhaps a gastroenterologist or neurologist—had already referred them to me because their tests had yielded no diagnosis.

After about two years of living in denial, many of these patients returned to me and told me they had finally followed my dietary advice, changed their diet and brought their symptoms under control. These follow-up visits made me feel pleased that my diagnosis helped them, yet I felt sad that they had wasted two years suffering illness.

Two Years of Distress

You may wonder why I can specify that they returned "after about two years." I can set this time interval because so many patients reacted to the aging food chemicals that the "some" who refused the diagnosis became *many*. I noticed that it invariably took this group about two years of suffering before accepting the diagnosis and returning to me to seek the care that brought them relief.

I mentioned this group of patients because I want to stress that reversing my patients' mental deterioration or reversing other distresses like restoring sensation to their feet and legs means they needed to limit their intake of foods they love. Please understand—because it affects so many people—if you suffer symptoms that these food chemicals might cause, they probably *do* cause them. I want to warn you: Do not deny the possibility that you might have to change your diet. Instead, you should embrace the chance that a diet change can bring your symptoms under control and lead you to better health.

Different Lactose Sensitivities

Several conditions can cause patients to suffer temporary lactose sensitivity, including celiac disease, a viral infection of the intestine, Crohn's disease, inflammation of the intestine, irritable bowel syndrome, or significant trauma to the intestines, including abdominal surgery. We are not discussing these diseases. Patients suffering from any of these other issues must follow the advice of their family doctors, internists, pediatricians, gastroenterologists, or other medical specialists—not the advice in this book. The sensitivity we are discussing is caused by the diet, advancing age or genetic makeup.

Genetics of Lactose Sensitivity

The lactose sensitivity we discuss—late-onset and not complicated by any of the above conditions—afflicts millions. Studies have identified the cause as changes in a gene, LCT, that allow us to absorb and use lactose. The LCT gene instructs cells to make the enzyme lactase, which splits lactose. The human intestinal tract cannot absorb lactose until the two sugars that make up the lactose molecule, glucose and galactose, are separated by the lactase enzyme. Lactase acts like a tiny man who pounds a wedge between the two sugar molecules of lactose, forcing them apart so we can digest them separately.

As most of us age, another gene, MCM6, progressively slows LCT's action. It acts like a switch that throttles down LCT's power to digest lactose, significantly lowering our ability to absorb and use lactose. This weakening of our lactose digestion is why my lactose-sensitive patients can only drink about four ounces of lactose-containing milk each day without symptoms.

It is easy to see why babies need the lactase enzyme to absorb and use large amounts of lactose-containing milk. If they lose their mother's milk from the mother's death or her inability to produce breast milk, they could become severely malnourished if they could not use a human breast milk substitute such as lactose-containing cow's milk.

Races of people who have raised cattle and consumed cow's milk as adults for thousands of years—for example, people of northern European backgrounds—can digest lactose as adults. This continued ability to use cow's milk occurs because of mutations in the genes that allow the consumption and metabolism of lactose. However, people whose ancestors as adults did not drink cow's milk—for example, people of African, Asian, Arab, Jewish, Greek, Italian, Hispanic, and American Indian backgrounds—commonly as adults lose much of their ability to digest lactose.

This ability to tolerate large amounts of lactose in races of people from cattle-herding countries must eventually weaken with age. I noticed that my aged patients of every background became unable to tolerate lactose. Many people survive with intact minds into their 90s and 100s; it would be interesting to know if they came from cattle-raising races.

Lactose Sensitivity Teaches Us About Sensitivity to the Aging Chemicals

My experience with patients sensitive to the aging chemicals showed me that lactose sensitivity is attached to these chemicals like a link is attached to a chain. It also taught me that lactose sensitivity usually precedes sensitivity to other food chemicals, including gluten, MSG, refined sugar, citrus acids, and LCSs. If food chemical sensitivity were a marching band, lactose would be in front swinging the baton.

Symptoms of Lactose Sensitivity

People sensitive to the troubling food chemicals share some symptoms such as tiredness and simply not feeling well. Each also has symptoms specific to the individual food chemical. Lactose intolerance has its symptoms, caused by undigested lactose in the intestines, leading to gas buildup. The gas forms because, as sensitive people age, the lactase enzyme that breaks apart the two sugars of lactose can no longer handle a large load of lactose. The undigested lactose then passes through the small intestine without being absorbed by the last part of the intestine, the large intestine.

In the large intestine, lactose meets live bacteria fully capable of digesting it. Unfortunately, bacterial digestion produces large volumes of gas and irritates the intestine. Within thirty minutes to two hours after drinking too much milk, people with lactose sensitivity can suffer stomach cramps and diarrhea. These two symptoms, gas and diarrhea, point to the diagnosis of lactose sensitivity. The abdominal cramping suggests that the digestion of lactose by bacteria in the large intestine stimulates the nerves that cause abdominal cramping.

The associated gas production is no slight problem. It can be voluminous and smelly. I know because I am lactose sensitive, and it is no fun evaluating patients while suffering this symptom in a small exam room. I am embarrassed to confess this symptom, but I feel I must. I want you to remember that I suffer from sensitivity to these food chemicals that age us, including lactose sensitivity. This sensitivity gives me a unique insight into the syndrome, increasing my ability to describe it to you and making me determined to tell you about it.

Treatment of Lactose Sensitivity (Lactase Deficiency)

I consider milk, with its content of calcium, valuable in the diet. Nature does, too. Some studies strongly point to the beneficial effects of milk: They show that adults who can drink milk are healthier and better able to have descendants to pass on these lactose-tolerant genes. Perhaps the improved health comes from the increased calcium from the dairy products they tolerate.

Over thousands of years, this genetic advantage has resulted in the races I mentioned having large numbers of members who, as adults, are tolerant of lactose.

However, some recent studies indicate that, in some adults, drinking cow's milk may not be healthy. Further studies should eventually confirm or deny this possibility. At the same time, any super-pasteurized milk can have too much MSG for many people because the breakdown of milk proteins during pasteurization frees glutamic acid that then becomes MSG. Further, although there are milk substitutes, including soymilk, yogurt, and cheese, they contain—or may contain—high quantities of MSG imparted to the milk during processing.

There are steps you can take if you must limit your intake of lactose-containing milk. First, consult with your doctor or a dietician. Read the information available on the internet, but be aware that there also is a lot of incorrect information there. Do not exceed your tolerance for lactose-containing milk. Be careful of milk made from other foods that may have excess MSG from processing. Ask your doctor or dietician if you should supplement your diet with calcium. Eat calcium-containing foods (dark, leafy greens like spinach, kale, turnips greens, or collard greens) if you tolerate these foods.

The Reason Lactose Is an Aging Chemical

I finally found that lactose belongs among the aging chemicals: It fits them well. Combining glucose and D-galactose forms lactose. We tolerate glucose well, absorb it, and use it to provide energy. We more poorly handle galactose. In 2010,

Dr. Kodeeswaran Parameswara, Department of Pathobiology, College of Veterinary Medicine, Auburn University, Alabama, stated, "Accumulating evidence suggests that mitochondrial dysfunction and oxidative stress play major roles in aging. Chronic administration of D-galactose has been reported to cause deterioration of cognitive and motor skills that are similar to symptoms of aging and, therefore, is regarded as a model of accelerated aging."

Scientists studying aging in animals are using this chronic administration of D-galactose to age animal brains. Since damage and aging of the brain cause dementia, I worry about feeding D-galactose to people with dementia. Unfortunately, D-galactose enriched foods are already in the diet, including avocado, cheese, cherries, celery, chocolate, honey, milk, kiwi, peanut, plums, and yogurt. Milk and its products have the most significant amount of D-galactose. Could there be a food chemical more suited to being classified among the "aging chemicals" sugar, MSG, and citrus acids?

What Lactose-Intolerant Patients Taught Me

I am grateful for the many lactose-sensitive patients whose insight into their condition taught me much about lactose sensitivity and its relation to the aging chemicals. They taught me that the coexistence of lactose sensitivity and sensitivity to the aging chemicals in so many patients indicates that lactose belongs to the same group of problem-causing chemicals. Lactose's stimulation of the intestine's nerves causing cramps and diarrhea suggests that, in sensitive people, lactose causes intestinal nerve irritation. Nerve irritation is a characteristic of the aging chemicals.

10

Managing Nerve-Related Disease

I have concentrated on the adverse effects of eating and drinking MSG, LCSs, gluten, refined sugar, citric acid, and lactose. These chemicals are neurotoxins when consumed in excess of what we tolerate. Why should that worry you? Because, in excess, these chemicals are systemic poisons.

They poison all of the body, especially the most essential system, the nervous system, which controls our activity, thoughts, and lives. We cannot function to the height of our abilities if our nervous system is damaged. And we cannot live if the damage is too severe. That's why you should worry.

This damage to our nervous systems from the neurotoxins in our diet is a significant cause of many diseases, of which the conditions below are examples:

- Alzheimer's disease
- Diabetes and diabetic neuropathy
- Mild cognitive impairment
- Parkinson's disease
- Huntington's disease

- Multiple sclerosis
- Amyotrophic lateral sclerosis
- Stroke
- Heart attacks
- Migraine headaches

Also, many other illnesses and disease conditions.

Diet changes are not the only treatments for the illnesses I discuss; your medical caregiver can provide other treatment methods and drugs to help you. However, those afflicted by a disease caused by food chemicals that damage and kill nerves should not consume the excess chemicals that become neurotoxins. In this book, *Escape from Dementia,* I stress diet changes that reversed my dementia and might also reverse your disease.

Now that you know more about the food chemicals that age us, you can see why I refer to them as "aging." As we grow older, we become more sensitive to these food chemicals: They drive this aging into us like a hammer drives a nail into wood. Limiting these chemicals is like putting down the hammer. If we do not cautiously select our foods and drinks, they will continue to injure and destroy the nerves controlling thinking, memory, balance, and other essential bodily functions. This nerve destruction increases the deterioration we experience with advancing years. As we limit our consumption of troubling foods and beverages, we limit dementia and slow the disabilities that accompany aging.

Our modern American diet promotes this aging and disease: Changing our diets can reverse this horrible deterioration. And I do mean "horrible deterioration." What else would you call a disease that damages the brain and turns the sufferer into a pitiful creature?

Alzheimer's Disease

I have suffered the mental deterioration of Alzheimer's disease. In this chapter, I started with this disease because it is the most common dementia, and it is my dementia. In Alzheimer's disease, the aging chemicals injure and ultimately destroy the nerves essential to retaining our thoughts and memories. They can, and do, change an independent and valuable member of society into a baby-like dependent of little use in our modern world.

The National Institute on Aging identifies early symptoms of Alzheimer's as memory loss, getting lost in traveling, taking longer to do daily tasks, and experiencing difficulty speaking, reading, writing, and adding and subtracting numbers (Alzheimer's Disease Fact Sheet, 2015). These symptoms affect me whenever I overindulge in these troubling food chemicals.

The Alzheimer's Association lists one of the warning signs of Alzheimer's as new problems with words in speaking or writing. They explain: "People with Alzheimer's may have trouble following or joining a conversation. They may stop in the middle of a conversation and have no idea how to continue, or they may repeat themselves. They may struggle with vocabulary, have problems finding the right word or call things by the wrong name (e.g., calling a 'watch' a 'hand-clock')" (*10 Early Signs and Symptoms of Alzheimer's*, 2016).

I suffered these symptoms; I had exceeded my tolerance of the aging chemicals and my speech became halting and

I could not finish sentences. Even today, my vocabulary and speech worsen if I am not cautious in the foods and drinks I choose. Dementia will reclaim me if I neglect my diet.

Prevention/Treatment of Alzheimer's Disease

I often think of a simple story that, to me, points to the treatment of Alzheimer's disease:

Three men bought new houses with wooden siding, and each painted his home, the first man with expensive and strongly protective paint, the second and third with progressively cheaper paints. To keep their houses scrupulously clean, each, once or twice daily, sprayed the house with an acid bath. The first house, painted with the best paint, showed no damage from the spray after eighty years. After fifty years, the less-protecting paint on the second house showed mild paint pitting and loss of luster from the acid spray. With the least protective, cheapest paint, the third house showed such severe damage from the spray; after forty years, it was completely uninhabitable.

In this story, we are the houses; the acid sprays are the neurotoxins we eat daily, and the paints protecting the homes are the genes that protect us from these diet chemicals. Some of us are lucky and, like the first home, our genes act like expensive paint; they protect us from the neurotoxins that harm others. We are the older people who are still driving cars and enjoying a sound mind at ninety years of age. Some of us are like the second homes protected by the less-expensive paints. Our genes only partially protect us; they allow our mental decline to become noticeable at about forty to sixty years of age and death sometime later. Some of us are like the third house that the acid washes completely devastated; incompetent genes fail us entirely, and we suffer harm and death from our diet at a younger age.

You may be asking yourself: "Why do those homeowners use an acid spray to clean their homes?" It is because they do not realize how much harm the spray can cause. We eat neurotoxins like refined sugar, LCSs, citric acid, and MSG for the same reason: We do not realize how much harm they cause. Or if we recognize this harm, we do not acknowledge it.

How do our homeowners stop the deterioration of their homes? They stop spraying them with acid washes. How do we prevent (or slow) the decline of our minds? We stop eating and drinking foods and beverages with excessive levels of these aging food chemicals.

Is it silly for me to use an example where owners spray their homes with acids? Yes! They should never have started. Is it silly for us to eat and drink foods containing neurotoxins? Yes! We should never have started.

Injury and death of nerve cells characterize Alzheimer's disease. To prevent further deterioration and reverse the decline, people with Alzheimer's disease should consume a diet that contains only as much of the aging chemicals as they can tolerate without further nerve damage.

Diabetes and Diabetic Neuropathy

Until the past few years, most doctors recognized only two types of diabetes: type 1 and type 2. Type 1 diabetes is also called "juvenile" or "insulin-dependent" diabetes, usually starting before thirty years of age and affecting a small but significant percentage of people with diabetes who must take insulin daily. Type 2 or "non-insulin dependent" diabetics affects ninety to ninety-five percent of the 26 million Americans with diabetes, who may or may not need to take insulin. Now, evidence is accumulating that Alzheimer's disease is also a type of diabetes. The Alzheimer's Association in *Diabetes and Cognitive Decline* (2015) discusses this new condition and complicated condition.

Complications of Diabetes

Many people with diabetes suffer significant nerve injury. Any nerve can be affected. Diabetes typically impacts the extremities. There, peripheral neuropathy (nerve damage) causes numbness and tingling in the feet and legs and can lead to muscle weakness and significant pain in the arms and legs, as well as loss of feeling and sensation. Significant balance problems and falling make the afflicted use walkers and wheelchairs. Bruising, broken bones, and further loss of feeling in the extremities can lead to amputation from injuries and infections.

Much of this damage arises from high levels of blood sugar. High blood sugar also harm diabetics' blood vessels, hearts, gastrointestinal systems, and renal systems.

Alzheimer's Disease Is Related to Diabetes

Today, throughout the world, about 35 million people have Alzheimer's disease. As the population ages, by 2050, this number can be expected to rise to 100 million. The potential number of people with memory disorders is overwhelming. The cost of treating this epidemic is already overwhelming.

For years, medical scientists knew that type 2 diabetics

were two to three times more likely to suffer Alzheimer's-related dementia than non-diabetics. The obese are similarly more likely to suffer Alzheimer's than the non-obese. Obesity and insulin resistance are features of the aging food chemicals, especially the excess refined sugar that we already discussed. The correlation between diabetes and Alzheimer's is strong, suggesting that diabetes predisposes its sufferers to Alzheimer's disease.

Resisting Alzheimer's Disease, Diabetes, and Diabetic Neuropathy
If a person is genetically susceptible to diabetes—and that genetic susceptibility is widespread as judged by the large numbers of people with diabetes—years of repeated consumption of the aging food chemicals can awaken a monster, the insulin resistance that characterizes diabetes. Combining obesity from fructose sugar with nerve damage caused by MSG and citrus acids launches a horrific nerve attack capable of bringing Alzheimer's disease and diabetes.

Prevention/Treatment of Diabetes
With nerve cell injury and nerve death characterizing this disease, persons susceptible to or in the early stages of diabetes should avoid foods containing large amounts of these food chemicals that age us, especially refined sugar with its fructose.

Mild Cognitive Impairment

People with mild cognitive impairment (MCI) suffer memory or other thought-related problems but are not as disabled as those with Alzheimer's disease. Unfortunately, as they age, many of these people progress to Alzheimer's disease.

Prevention/Treatment of Mild Cognitive Impairment

Studies show a relationship between diabetes and MCI. Refined sugar is a cause—or aggravating factor—in diabetes, and people suffering MCI should strictly avoid excess refined sugar and the other neurotoxins. After all, it makes no sense to feed people with MCI foods and beverages containing increased amounts of the aging chemicals.

Parkinson's Disease

This disease occurs due to the death of specific cells in the brain that produce dopamine. Dopamine is a neurotransmitter—as is glutamic acid—by which nerve cells send signals to other nerve cells. With the decrease in dopamine, muscle activity is affected, resulting in shaking, rigidity, slowness of movement, and difficulty walking and keeping an even gait. Often, cognitive and behavioral problems can occur, which can progress, in advanced stages, to dementia.

Prevention/Treatment of Parkinson's Disease

Genetic causes are known or suspected in a subset of people with Parkinson's disease. However, whether or not a known gene deficiency causes Parkinson's disease, nerve cell injury and death characterize this disease. I believe it makes no sense to feed people with Parkinson's disease foods and beverages with excess troubling food chemicals and take the chance that these foods and drinks increase their nerve injury.

Huntington's Disease

Huntington's disease (formerly known as Huntington's chorea) is a genetic disorder that involves the death of nerve cells throughout the brain—but most prominently in the area of the brain called the basal ganglia; these cells play a crucial role in movement and behavior control. The term "chorea" refers to a disorder involving brief, repetitive, jerky, involuntary movement. As this disease progresses, the sufferer's cognitive abilities progressively diminish.

Prevention/Treatment of Huntington's Disease

Because it is best to limit our diet-inflicted destruction of nerve cells, it is best to avoid excess aging food chemicals.

Multiple Sclerosis

Multiple sclerosis (MS) is a disease caused by the body's immune system attacking the central nervous system (including the brain, spinal cord, and optic nerves). This central nervous system sustains the most damage. Myelin, the protective fatty/protein coat wrapping around the nerves' axons, is injured ("axons" are the projections from the nerves that reach other nerve cells).

Through its effect on nerves, MS can impact almost every body system, including eyesight, muscles, sensation, and the autonomic nervous system. Damage to the autonomic nervous system can cause urinary incontinence, constipation, erectile dysfunction, vaginal dryness, hypotension, irregular heartbeat, and other symptoms. (It also promotes the disease dysautonomia). The location in the nervous system where MS damages neurons determines the symptoms experienced.

Prevention/Treatment of Multiple Sclerosis
Because nerve cell injury and nerve death characterize this illness, sufferers with MS should avoid foods with excess aging food chemicals.

Amyotrophic Lateral Sclerosis

In amyotrophic lateral sclerosis, also known as "ALS" or "Lou Gehrig's disease," the progressive destruction in the brain and spinal cord of the nerves that control muscle action can eventually lead to total paralysis. The inherited form of this disease arises from mutated genes, although other genes may also be involved. One theory suggests the immune system probably participates in the destruction of these nerves, as does the mishandling of protein in nerve cells.

Prevention/Treatment of Amyotrophic Lateral Sclerosis
Most sufferers have higher glutamic acid (MSG) levels in the spinal fluid around the nerve cells. If you recall our discussion of MSG, you can understand why, with nerve cell impairment characterizing this disease, sufferers should avoid consuming excess aging chemicals.

Migraine Headaches

As we discussed earlier, I found that the aging food chemicals are a significant cause of painful migraine headaches among my patients.

Prevention/Treatment of Migraine Headaches
We already discussed migraine headaches. With nerve and artery irritation causing migraine headache pain, sufferers

should avoid foods and beverages with excess aging food chemicals.

A Clarification

Please be aware that I do not attribute the causes of these various diseases only to foods. I tried specifying some of the other reasons, many known and many only suspected, including the involvement of our genes. If genes that limit damage from these diet chemicals continued to work well, we would never suffer these diseases; they could not trouble us. Unfortunately, we must suffer these diseases. Once they are recognized, we should follow a treatment that slows their progress. That means being cautious of our diet.

Changing the Basic Course of Diseases

Changing the basic course of these diseases may be possible. Not by changing the genes that allow them; we can't do that, but we can take on these genes' tasks. Medical studies show how to slow the onset of these diseases; my experience shows that they can be stopped and even reversed. The following is an example of one method I noticed among my patients that showed how they could be slowed, stopped, and reversed.

I used injections to treat many patients for their allergies to house dust, mold, and pollen. It became apparent to me that the injections had a remarkable effect on my patients' immune systems. As long as the injections contained house dust, they quieted the hyperactive immune system that causes allergies. Not only did the allergic shots quiet down symptoms like severe hay fever and asthma, but they also calmed symptoms of autoimmune diseases like lupus and MS.

Autoimmune diseases like lupus and MS frequently cause symptom flares, worsening the autoimmune disease, each flare leading to worse debility. Stopping these periods of worsening should—and in my patients did—slow the progression of the autoimmune disease. It reduced or eliminated these flares; the injection treatment (which I was using for allergies) prevented the deterioration of flares. The autoimmune disease did not seem to worsen as long as the injection treatment continued.

I am not urging you to seek allergy injection treatments, but I wanted to show you that with various treatments, we can resist the progression of diseases, even autoimmune diseases. Diet changes also provides much resistance to these diseases in many people, witness my dementias and the many diseases suffered by my patients.

Autoimmune and Damaged Nerve Diseases

How much help can you expect from avoiding the aging food chemicals? You can expect significant benefit if you suffer from deteriorating nerves. Consider, again, my illustration of the three houses and their paint:

The house with the excellent paint had no deterioration, similar to the people who are not susceptible to nerve deterioration. They do not need to avoid these food chemicals. The following two houses experienced a decline from less-protective paint, similar to people suffering nerve damage and nerve death from the aging chemicals. Avoiding them can help you fight against nerve deterioration, much like stopping the acid wash would help prevent the houses from deteriorating.

And, to make this treatment even more enticing, I am convinced that we who suffer nerve deterioration can regain the ability to remember, plan, and tie our shoes. We can live independently. Further, we can make this diet change at home. The earlier we start the diet, the better.

On the other hand, if we continue to eat and drink excessive amounts of the chemicals that age us, the damage may become irreversible. Remember that the acid washes damaged the last house so badly that it was not habitable. That house is like the severely damaged patients who need the care provided by memory units in health care settings. They should have reduced their exposure to the aging chemicals long before sinking so profoundly into the disease.

With careful dietary practices, we should avoid this outcome. We can alter the progression of Alzheimer's disease, Lou Gehrig's disease, Parkinson's disease, and other diseases for many years. There is even a good chance that we can reverse much of the damage! We only need to try!

Why Did I Keep Repeating Prevention/Treatment Advice?

Repetition is good for memory. Because the advice is the same in so many diseases, I hope repetition of this dietary avoidance plants this advice so deeply in your mind that you remember it. Repetition may help you realize that we damage more than the brain by this whole-body poisoning by these food chemicals. The troubling chemicals poison millions of people not only in our country but worldwide. Treating these people while feeding them our poisonous diet is only minimally effective and can bankrupt our country. We must spread the news that many of those afflicted with the dementias can resist and recover from these diseases in their own homes at own their dining tables.

11
Cautions and Notes

We discussed the aging chemicals separately. Now I want to discuss them as a group. I will review some of the information I gave you and add some new information to help you better understand this food sensitivity and its treatment. I will also propose and answer some questions that probably occurred to you as we discussed the aging food chemicals.

As we discussed, the aging food chemicals are also the chemicals that activate our taste buds—in short, the foods that harm us taste good. They damage and even kill nerves in our body and brain.

When to Avoid These Chemicals

Should everyone avoid or limit consumption of the foods and beverages that contain excesses of the aging food chemicals? There are two answers to that question.

The First Answer

Yes, everybody—even those free of the symptoms of nerve damage and destruction—should avoid these foods and beverages. Years of silent nerve destruction pass before the sufferer notices this damage; that's why avoiding these chemicals is appropriate even when no deterioration is noticeable. I believe this is the correct answer, but I realize that it is not a realistic answer. These food chemicals taste good and make meals tasty; without them, a meal can taste flat. I admit that few people will avoid these foods and beverages if they have not noticed signs of mental deterioration, whether it be the inability to feel their feet, memory defects, difficulty talking or other signs of nerve damage.

The Second Answer

Suppose you have a family history of Alzheimer's disease, Lou Gehrig's disease, diabetic loss of sensation in the legs and feet, or other diseases of nerve degeneration. In that case, you should avoid these foods and beverages to decrease your chance of suffering the same conditions that troubled other members of your family.

If you notice nerve damage in yourself or your loved ones, you should feel so threatened that you will take any available measures to fight off these tragic diseases.

Medical caregivers may tell that, from your family history, you or a loved one have a genetic potential to suffer nerve disease. If they do, or if tests indicate that you have a hereditary predisposition toward these diseases, avoiding these chemicals may prevent or at least slow the onset and progress of nerve deterioration.

I have visions of wandering through memory care units and finding them empty. I believe this will happen and that strict avoidance of excess aging food chemicals will help empty these wards. That is why I write.

How Strictly to Avoid These Foods

Again, there are several answers. If you or your loved one shows nerve damage symptoms—especially mental deterioration—strictly avoid foods and beverages with excess amounts of these chemicals. As repeatedly discussed here, aging food chemicals are not harmful if consumed in small quantities. After all, they are vital constituents of the body. We can consume limited amounts of these chemicals without apparent harm, especially in the young. However, as we age and nerve damage progresses, cautious use of the aging food chemicals has a chance to reverse the symptoms. When numbness and tingling of the extremities or increasing difficulty remembering the previous day's events or other signs of nerve disease appear, we must realize that we are failing. Do not hide this failure from yourself or a loved one. Then, to fight this deterioration, we must reduce our intake of these troubling chemicals.

Should We Start Avoiding These Chemicals Early in Life?

Yes, absolutely, we should. But, practically, how many of us will deny ourselves the incredible luxury of an MSG-flavored steak; who will rob our children of that delightful fructose-packed ice cream cone?

Only when we become frightened enough for our future, or that of a loved one, will we completely change our diets.

How Long Do Foods Remain in the Body?

From my experiences and those of my patients, foods remain in the body for about three days. If, during a meal, you have consumed an unwise amount of the troubling food chemicals, be especially careful to reduce your consumption of these chemicals for at least three days to let them leave your body.

Is This Diet Too Difficult to Follow?

No, not at all when you consider its benefits. You desperately want to stop nerve disease. Even beyond that, you want to recover from these symptoms—you want to return to thinking clearly, to talking freely, to slowing down your shaking. Along with lifestyle changes, these diet changes should help your damaged nerves recover. Do not think of this avoidance as difficult; think of it as hopeful. Be hopeful that you can continue to feel—or return to feeling—normal through avoiding excesses of these aging food chemicals. You will also lose some of the frailties you thought were caused by your age; you have a significant chance of becoming biologically younger.

The Brain Recovers Its Ability to Think and Plan

Doctors used to think that brain damage was irreversible. It is not! Both the brain and peripheral nerves can recover. The most dramatic proof of this recovery is in the field of "face transplants." Nerves from the transplanted face unite with the underlying tissue and the brain learns to use these nerves to animate the face. More proof concerns learning a new skill; the part of the brain learning this new skill enlarges as you learn the skill. It is even possible that the damage to your brain that put the cane in your hand or sat you in a wheelchair can be repaired or taken over by another part of the brain if you will only stop killing the baby nerves trying to reach and repair your brain.

The brain is a living organ capable of repairing itself

unless something you eat and drink prevents this repair. Yes, the brain can learn and adapt.

Avoiding the Aging Chemicals Is Not Enough

No. It would be best if you had other treatments. In this book, we concentrate on dietary chemicals you should avoid in your quest to slow or reverse mental deterioration. Other measures such as physical and mental exercise also help in slowing and repairing nerve destruction.

With these thoughts, I end this portion of this book about diet disease and how it may cause distressing nerve deterioration. As you try to avoid the foods I discussed, I hope that these diet changes bring you control of your disease. I further hope that they guide you to a return of the health and youth these troubling food chemicals took from you.

12

Diet and Disease

In this chapter, the rubber meets the road. If you or a loved one have dementia, you need to know the foods and beverages to avoid or include in your diet. The modern American diet contains these destructive aging chemicals, sugar (fructose), MSG, citrus acids, and lactose, all combining to age us. It is their excess that we poorly tolerate; smaller amounts we handle well. Many of our familiar vegetables and fruits contain these chemicals in excessive amounts, and they tempt our nerves of taste, prompting us to buy and eat them. Their ability to harm us forces us to avoid these fruits and vegetables or prepare them in ways that reduce their concentration.

If it tastes sweet, robust, or fruity, it probably has excess sugar, MSG, lactose, or citrus acids. That includes many manufactured products, including sweet, carbonated beverages, extra delicious-tasting meat, and fruity foods and beverages. A breakfast of sugar cereal, a lunch of pizza, and a between-meal snack of yogurt followed by a dinner of sausage with a dessert of key lime pie and ice cream will lead the dementia-sensitive consumer into dementia. Especially if your meals are accompanied by milk.

The diet for mildly and moderately afflicted people with

dementias is simple, but the multiplicity of aging chemicals and the variety of possible symptoms they cause made it challenging to determine which foods and beverages to limit or avoid. In seeking to identify these foods and beverages, I have spent years determining which of the varied components of our diet increase my dementia. We eat many foods daily, and as I check one food or beverage an unappreciated troubling food can alter results and I must constantly beware of this possibility; sometimes, I must repeat the test because I feel the results are uncertain. It can take days and even weeks to examine one food or beverage.

The results I present are as good as I could make them. As I continue to test foods and beverages, I will be able to recheck many of these foods and I will keep you informed of the results in future books. I feel confident that the diet advice I present here can be used by people with Alzheimer's, Parkinson's, Lewy body, and other dementias and all the other non-dementia diseases like strokes, obesity, and heart attacks, which are also heavily influenced, even caused, by our diet.

I look forward to the time when other sufferers will follow this diet and reverse their dementia. Then we can compare notes on which foods and beverages we tolerate.

You Must Cautiously Choose Your Diet

Many times, what we should eat or avoided is not apparent. An incident that happened to me helps illustrate this point. It was during a two-day trip to see the beautiful fall colors of Minnesota. Only it became a one-day trip because I ate a buffet dinner at a restaurant at a charming resort. I thought I could eat this one dinner without reacting to the food chemicals the chef might have been using: I asked my server to be sure that my foods be free of seasonings and condiments. I ate only the salad greens, no dressing, and a small steak. That night I slept poorly, perhaps only two hours of light, non-refreshing sleep. I suspected that food chemicals flavoring the meat caused this poor sleep. I knew that I couldn't trust the food in this lovely restaurant and needed to return home to my own cooking or my symptoms, including sleep deprivation, would worsen. I came home the next day, the same day that I experienced abdominal distress.

I typically react to excess MSG flavoring in my meal with poor sleep and abdominal distress, so these symptoms confirmed my suspicions that I reacted to the MSG in my meal. Further corroborating my suspicions: When I ate the meat, it had the delicious flavor of MSG. This experience reinforced my desire to tell whoever will listen to avoid a similar experience by, if at all possible, preparing their own meals.

The trip was not a waste of time. The trees were beautiful. I gave a discussion about reactions to the food chemicals, in which I pointed out the foods and beverages to eat and those to avoid. The audience reacted well to my presentation, and afterword several people told me the talk was great! I was so pleased with their comments; they made the trip worthwhile.

My Experience With the Diet

Perhaps you will better understand the diet if I tell you how I follow it. By now, you know that Alzheimer's disease severely affects me and has affected me for many years, and I also experience some characteristics of Parkinson's disease, a not unusual combination. Avoiding eating and drinking excessive amounts of the aging chemicals allows me to recover from this dementia, although I still suffer some memory loss; my memory is gradually improving and is better than it has been in the past. If I return to excess consumption of these chemicals, dementia symptoms return; fear of this return keeps me true to the diet (at least mainly faithful to the diet, I do cheat at times). My treatment of my dementia by a cautious diet should help guide others who suffer from sensitivity to these chemicals.

Cookbooks, the internet, and your experience in food preparation brought you much information on food preparation. My purpose is to provide an overview of food preparation, to tell you why you should follow the diet I have developed. Repeating here what you already know or can learn elsewhere would extend this chapter unnecessarily.

A Reward for the Cautious Diet

Sufferers with dementia may feel depressed about being forced to avoid many foods and beverages they love—foods and beverages with the marked sweetness, robustness, and fruitiness conferred by high levels of sugar, lactose, MSG, and citrus acids. They can cheer up! Years of eating and drinking large amounts of these chemicals have battered their nerves of taste so severely that the subtle natural flavor of foods and beverages not loaded with these chemicals seem almost tasteless. These tastes can recover and allow enjoyment of foods if we avoid the chemicals long enough for the nerves to recover from this beating, perhaps within two to six months. Further, the ability to taste becomes better with each succeeding month. This natural taste is enjoyable and will reward us for our efforts.

Caution

If you know you react to certain foods or beverages, even if I indicate that they are acceptable, do not eat or drink them.

The Search for a Healthy Diet

The Mediterranean, DASH, and MIND diets delay the onset of Alzheimer's dementia: They are healthy diets. Even though they are good diets, delay the onset of diseases including dementia, and help sufferers of many diseases, they cannot reverse conditions such as dementia. Patients following these diets still die from these diseases. I believe they die because, although the diets stress avoidance of fructose sugar and somewhat avoid MSG, they do not stress avoiding excesses of the other harmful chemicals. Avoiding these excesses allowed me to recover from dementia, and I believe this same avoidance will enables many others to follow my path to recovery.

The Fat Regulatory System

I will review a healthy diet's impact on obesity to remind you why these diets are healthy. Healthy diets include much animal fat and vegetable oils such as olive oil. My diet is a high-fat diet, but as long as I avoid all sweet treats, my body does not absorb this excess fat and passes much of it into my stools, especially when I first followed the diet and as I continued to lose over one hundred pounds. Therefore, although my diet is a high-fat diet, at first it prevented me from absorbing much fat.

Now that I have reached the weight my body desires, I do absorb fat, but my weight stays at or below 140 pounds. At night, my body burns off the excess fat I accumulated during the day. I do not know if there is a name for this system in our bodies that regulates the amount of fat that remains in our bodies, so I named it the *fat regulatory system.* If I return to eating fructose-sweet treats, I poison this system: It stops working. My scale shows weight gain and obesity begins again.

Further, if I eat or drink food or beverages with fructose, my dementia symptoms worsen; my speech becomes broken as I hunt for words; my memory deteriorates for names, places, and things. In addition, I worry that I return to the possibility of suffering strokes and heart attacks caused by fat storage in the arteries to the heart and brain. I avoid these threatening conditions as much as possible; I avoid loading my diet with large amounts of fructose sugar.

Diet Response to Mild, Moderate, or Severe Disease

People who suffer minimal or no dementia symptoms should still be aware of the dangers that hide in our modern diet. Then they can choose to avoid foods and beverages with excess sugar, MSG, milk, and citrus acids that they can easily give up. Even if they do not experience mild symptoms of dementia, when they need highly functioning minds before engaging in a stressful life experience, perhaps before a test, work interview, or other stressful experiences, they could closely follow a cautious diet for at least a week. The diet change should significantly prepare their mind and body for the stressful event and increase their chance for a successful outcome. This suggestion becomes even more pertinent as mild dementia symptoms arise.

Diet Response to Mild to Moderate Dementia Symptoms

With *mild dementia symptoms,* reasonable diligence in reducing the intake of these dangerous chemicals should be sufficient to slow the progression of dementia. Still, the afflicted should be aware that with age, they become more sensitive to these food chemicals and their health can progressively deteriorate if they continue to consume more harmful chemicals than they tolerate that they tolerated earlier in life. Fear of mind and body deterioration should prompt the moderately symptomatic to reduce their intake of the dangerous foods and beverages, including some that they enjoy. As each person's diet preferences differs from every other person's, I can give no hard and fast rules that cover each person's diet choices. My readers and audiences should realize they must pursue a cautious diet with less sugar, MSG, lactose, or citrus acids. If they do not use their innate intelligence to change their diets, nature will destroy this intelligence. Nature is unforgiving. Beware!

Response to Severe Dementia Symptoms

Those with severe dementia symptoms should realize that nature points a loaded gun at us and shoots! This shot happens every time we eat and drink dangerous foods and beverages. We must unload the firearm and let our bodies repair the damage caused by the excess of harmful foods and drinks that are the bullets of this figurative gun. Avoid these excesses!

What symptoms should we look for when we suspect our dementia symptoms are entering the severe stage? We must acknowledge that dementia is no longer mild or moderate when certain events happen:

- We develop senile dementia (I believe this is treatable Alzheimer's disease).
- Our family takes away the keys to our car.
- We hunt for words instead of just saying them as they come into our minds.
- Your caretaker is preparing a place for you in a memory unit.
- You poorly remember relatives' and friends' names.
- You no longer remember to pay your bills.
- Your sleep, balance, hearing, sight, and other abilities deteriorate.
- You suffered a stroke, heart attack, diabetes, or other diet-caused diseases.

Does Severe Dementia Mean We Must Die of This Disease?

No, no, no, no, no! You or a loved one with severe dementia do not need to die of this disease. Adults in their 90s with intact minds show that age does not kill nerves; eating a poisonous diet for years kills nerves. The brain constantly refreshes itself at any age if our diet does not kill the immature nerves that refresh the brain. We simply need to change what we eat and drink to allow these new nerve cells to live, reach, and bring youth to the brain. I have had severe dementia for years and could not write this book if I, with my diet choices, had kept killing my baby nerve cells.

If diseases like obesity, stroke, autoimmune disorder and heart attack trouble you or a loved one, my diet is still the diet to follow because it avoids the foods and beverages that precipitate or worsen these conditions.

I often dream of patients on a memory unit following my diet. After a year on the diet I expect that up to half of them would leave the unit with competent, young minds repopulated with new nerve cells to enjoy life and live independently.

13

For the Mildly/ Moderately Afflicted

People with mild to moderate dementia tolerate vegetables, fruit, and the meat of animals, fowl, fish, and other seafood. We readily accept these foods in the early stages of dementia and can follow diets like the Mediterranean, MIND, and Mayo Clinic Diets. You must modify these diets as dementia becomes more severe and the afflicted transition from mild to moderate and then to severe dementia. The diet needs modification because the food chemicals that age us and that these diets advocate when our symptoms are mild need to be progressively reduced.

I mentioned that foods and beverages that taste sweet, robust, or fruity most likely contain excesses of these chemicals. We cannot live without these chemicals, we use them in our daily lives, but consuming excessive amounts turns healthy food chemicals into nerve toxins.

To emphasize this point, I will restate it: In mild dementia, the afflicted can consume all foods and beverages, even those containing excessive quantities of refined sugar, MSG, galactose, and citrus acids. Except (and there is always an "except") mild dementia may never transition to severe dementia if people susceptible to dementia significantly reduce consumption of these chemicals before symptoms begin or when it is first noticed. Further, the dementia may never progress to increased brain deterioration in the mildly symptomatic if these troubling chemicals are significantly avoided. These hopeful thoughts peek out from the results of research of the Mediterranean Diet that show us that avoiding excess refined sugar retards the advance of the dementias significantly. We can further advance these wonderful characteristics by limiting all the chemicals that age us, including fructose, MSG, galactose, and citrus acids. In my case, avoiding excesses of all these chemicals allowed me to crawl out of the muddy swamp of dementia, and I expect can similarly help others also escape this disease.

Even the mildly affected need to avoid any foods that they know trouble them.

As I discuss the diet for people minimally involved with dementia, I will tell you how this diet relates to the diet of the severely affected. You can decide if you will more stringently avoid the troubling foods and beverages to further advance the possibility that your dementia will stop and regress.

I have just described the rewards of following my diet if you have dementia. In other diet-caused disease like stroke, obesity, heart disease, depression, or autoimmune disorders, try the same diet change. Reducing the poison in your diet should help relieve any diseases and continuing to feed these diet toxins should make them worse.

Foods and Beverages to Use With Great Caution

Low-Calorie Sweeteners

I discussed this. We suffer dementia because we want foods and beverages that taste sweet, robust, and fruity. Why take a chance of eating and drinking chemicals with unusual powers to make our foods and beverages sweet, robust, or fruity, chemicals that assist the worsening of your dementia?

Alcoholic Beverages

The body treats alcoholic beverages like it treats fructose. It doesn't know what to do with them. I drink only small amounts of alcohol and realize it would be better if I avoided it altogether.

Healthy diets allow limited amounts of wine. However, I believe wine contains health dangers, including the acidity of the wine. We should avoid wine or, if consumed, do so during the meal, not when the stomach is empty. I suspect that too rapid absorption may promote more nerve damage than slow absorption. An occasional glass of wine may be acceptable during meals, but not every day. Wine worries me, and I believe it would be best to drink it only occasionally.

Meat

Unprocessed foods like beef, pork, chicken, turkey, fish, and seafood have some troubling chemicals that the mildly to moderately afflicted can eat without hesitation. These problematic chemicals become more worrisome for people with more severe dementia, and I will describe this further in my next book when describing the diet for the severely sensitive.

Avoiding processed foods such as soups, sausages and injected meats because of their content of troubling chemicals becomes more critical as dementia progresses from mild to moderate. At a restaurant, ask that the food be unseasoned and try to determine if the chef knows if it has been seasoned before being brought to the restaurant. Make sure the waiter communicates your request to the chef to avoid seasoning. Unfortunately, this request is often ineffective, and you eat seasoned meat.

Drippings

I experimented with drippings from meat and noticed a worsening of my dementia symptoms, suggesting that some chemical is freed from the cooked meat and concentrated in the drippings. (According to *Dictionary.com*, drippings are wax, fat, or other liquid produced from something by the effect of heat). I discard all drippings and avoid gravy. Although those with mild dementia can consume drippings, avoiding them may be the wiser decision.

Fats and Oils

Sugar, MSG, and citrus acids dissolve in water. Fats such as animal fat, butter, and oil like olive oil contain troubling chemicals because their foods contain these chemicals. However, these fats and oils are acceptable in mild to moderate dementia. Although fat from foods may be involved in such diseases as obesity, strokes, and heart attacks, current diet research points to carbohydrates (fructose) as far more potent causes of these diseases than the fat we eat. Research also suggests that a high-fat, low-carbohydrate diet is healthier than the reverse, a high-carbohydrate, low-fat diet. Still, I question the healthiness of a high-fat diet not combined with avoidance of fructose, MSG, milk, and citrus acids. In severe dementia, fats and oils become far more worrisome.

There is evidence that extra virgin olive oil has a dementia-sparing effect in laboratory animals and may have the same effect in humans with mild to moderate severity symptoms. Olive oil becomes worrisome as mild symptoms worsen to moderate and severe symptoms.

Fruit

Many fruits contain wonderful components that promote health, but many also contain fructose or citrus acids. With mild to moderate dementia, fruits should be acceptable in your diet. This changes as moderate dementia symptoms progress to severe. With my severe dementia, I regard fruit as candy and eat small amounts. Several times weekly, I include a small dish of blueberries as a treat in the afternoon. Choose the small berries called wild blueberries. The larger berries taste as if they contain excess fructose and citrus. I enjoy a pear on days when I do not eat blueberries.

Vegetables

With mild dementia, experts encourage us to include vegetables in our diets. As dementia worsens from mild to moderate, the diet becomes more restricted with vegetables and unprocessed meat the mainstays. It is best to select vegetables that lack a noticeable sweet or citrus taste. These acceptable vegetables include asparagus, beets, lettuce, kale, and squash. Some vegetables, such as beans, carrots, corn, potatoes, and yams, contain excess chemicals. In mild to moderate dementia, steaming or boiling the vegetables until soft seems to reduce this excess. I believe cooking the cabbage family until soft is best. I do not use salad dressing.

Beverages

Plain water is OK. Coffee and tea contain antioxidants and are considered healthy, low-calorie beverages. However, these beverages keep me awake at night, and I avoid them. Most fruit juices contain sugar and citrus acids and are acceptable in mild dementia but avoid them in moderate disease. Milk intolerance seems to accompany dementia, and I tolerate milk poorly. I do not drink milk or consume milk-derived products.

Salt

Salt in small quantities is acceptable. However, when I have consumed excessive amounts of the aging chemicals and feel bloated, consuming too much salt accentuates the bloating. I believe doing so is unhealthy and dangerous. To restate: I avoid consuming too much salt, especially if I stray from my diet and feel bloated and uncomfortable.

Goodbye for Now

I have given you enough information about our diet and disease that you should be aware of our diet's contribution to many diseases. There is much more to tell and I will give you more information in the second book of my *Retaining the Mind* series. If you know enough about the diet and disease and follow the path I took, you have a chance of preventing or recovering from many illnesses.

www.ingramcontent.com/pod-product-compliance
Lightning Source LLC
Chambersburg PA
CBHW061808250726
48657CB00001B/338